How to Conduct In-Person Interviews for Surveys

2nd edition

THE SURVEY KIT, Second Edition

Purposes: The purposes of this 10-volume Kit are to enable readers to prepare and conduct surveys and to help readers become better users of survey results. Surveys are conducted to collect information; surveyors ask questions of people on the telephone, face-to-face, and by mail. The questions can be about attitudes, beliefs, and behavior as well as socioeconomic and health status. To do a good survey, one must know how to plan and budget for all survey tasks, how to ask questions, how to design the survey (research) project, how to sample respondents, how to collect reliable and valid information, and how to analyze and report the results.

Users: The Kit is for students in undergraduate and graduate classes in the social and health sciences and for individuals in the public and private sectors who are responsible for conducting and using surveys. Its primary goal is to enable users to prepare surveys and collect data that are accurate and useful for primarily practical purposes. Sometimes, these practical purposes overlap with the objectives of scientific research, and so survey researchers will also find the Kit useful.

Format of the Kit: All books in the series contain instructional objectives, exercises and answers, examples of surveys in use and illustrations of survey questions, guidelines for action, checklists of dos and don'ts, and annotated references.

Volumes in The Survey Kit:

1. **The Survey Handbook, 2nd**
   Arlene Fink
2. **How to Ask Survey Questions, 2nd**
   Arlene Fink
3. **How to Conduct Self-Administered and Mail Surveys, 2nd**
   Linda B. Bourque and Eve P. Fielder
4. **How to Conduct Telephone Surveys, 2nd**
   Linda B. Bourque and Eve P. Fielder
5. **How to Conduct In-Person Interviews for Surveys, 2nd**
   Sabine Mertens Oishi
6. **How to Design Survey Studies, 2nd**
   Arlene Fink
7. **How to Sample in Surveys, 2nd**
   Arlene Fink
8. **How to Assess and Interpret Survey Psychometrics, 2nd**
   Mark S. Litwin
9. **How to Manage, Analyze, and Interpret Survey Data, 2nd**
   Arlene Fink
10. **How to Report on Surveys, 2nd**
    Arlene Fink

The Survey Kit 2ᵉᵈ

5

Sabine Mertens Oishi

How to Conduct In-Person Interviews for Surveys

2nd edition

THE SURVEY KIT
TSK 2

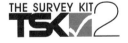

SAGE Publications
International Educational and Professional Publisher
Thousand Oaks ▪ London ▪ New Delhi

For information:

Sage Publications, Inc.
2455 Teller Road
Thousand Oaks, California 91320
E-mail: order@sagepub.com

Sage Publications Ltd.
6 Bonhill Street
London EC2A 4PU
United Kingdom

Sage Publications India Pvt. Ltd.
M-32 Market
Greater Kailash I
New Delhi 110 048 India

Printed in the United States of America

Library of Congress Cataloging-in-Publication Data

The survey kit.—2nd ed.
    p. cm.
Includes bibliographical references.
ISBN 0-7619-2510-4 (set : pbk.)
1. Social surveys. 2. Health surveys. I. Fink, Arlene.
HN29 .S724 2002
300'.723—dc21   2002012405

This book is printed on acid-free paper.

02 03 04 05 10 9 8 7 6 5 4 3 2 1

Acquisitions Editor:	C. Deborah Laughton
Editorial Assistant:	Veronica Novak
Copy Editor:	Judy Selhorst
Production Editor:	Diane S. Foster
Typesetter:	Bramble Books
Proofreader:	Cheryl Rivard
Cover Designer:	Ravi Balasuriya
Production Designer:	Michelle Lee

Contents

Acknowledgments

I am indebted to numerous thoughtful and dedicated individuals who have shared their expertise, wisdom, and examples from their work. Very special thanks are extended to Julia Anderson of the Center for Health Studies, Group Health Cooperative of Puget Sound, for sharing her vast knowledge of survey interviewing and for examples used to illustrate many points in this book. Many thanks also to the interviewers and supervisors of Project IMPACT (Improving Mood: Promoting Access to Collaborative Treatment), particularly Virginia Seguin Mika, whose real-life interviewing experiences and tips enriched my descriptions of what it takes to do the job. Thank you to Tonya Marmon for conversations that helped shape the chapter on data management and analysis.

I would also like to thank Patricia Harmon and John Dermand for sharing their supervisory expertise from many projects, as well as materials from which some of the examples in this book were derived, and Elena Reigadas, whose knowledge of cross-cultural and translation issues enriched my perspective greatly. My appreciation is also extended to Robert Haile for permission to adapt questionnaire and training materials from his projects, particularly the Kaiser/UCLA Sigmoidoscopy-Based Case-Control Study of Colon Polyps (Sigmoid Study), and to James H. Frey for fruitful collaboration on a previous edition covering both telephone and in-person interviewing.

Very special thanks go to Jürgen Unützer for permission to include materials from Project IMPACT in some of the examples in this book, and for creating a work opportunity that has provided me with a tremendous learning experience.

I would like to extend special appreciation to Arlene Fink for support, learning, and examples derived from shared survey experiences. Thanks also go to C. Deborah Laughton of Sage Publications for encouragement and support, to several anonymous reviewers whose constructive suggestions helped round out the final draft of the manuscript, and to Haneefa Wawda for formatting assistance.

How to Conduct In-Person Interviews for Surveys: Learning Objectives

The aim of this book is to guide you in the preparation and administration of in-person **survey** interviews. Its specific objectives are to prepare you to do the following:

- Describe the advantages and disadvantages of the use of in-person interviews compared with telephone and self-administered surveys

- Discuss the administrative considerations involved in setting up a project involving in-person interviews

- Write interview questions with structured interviewer instructions

- Distinguish programmer instructions from interviewer instructions for computer-assisted interviews

- Construct useful visual aids

- Organize a flowing interview script that considers possible question-order effects

- Write an informative introductory statement

- Write a preletter

- Write a script for a precall

- Design an eligibility screen

- Write and appropriately place transition statements

- Understand the informed consent process and how to apply it

- Write a job description for an interviewer

- Develop an interviewer training manual

- Deal with interview refusal attempts

- Establish the environment for an in-person interview

- Record responses and correct errors in paper and computer-assisted interviews

- Design an interviewer training session

- Describe the role of a supervisor

- Understand the process of data cleaning

- Describe differences in quantitative and qualitative interview styles

- Describe cultural considerations involved in in-person interviews

- Understand issues related to the translation of interviews into other languages

1

Overview: The Five Ws— Who? What? When? Where? Why?

An in-person interview is a purposeful conversation between participants who are physically in the same place. Interviewer and respondent are present to one another in ways that are not possible in telephone-administered, computer-administered, or self-administered surveys. In-person interviewing, also called *face-to-face* or *personal interviewing*, takes many forms and has many uses. Reporters interview people to gain information for news stories. Doctors interview patients to gather clues to help make diagnoses. Employers interview job applicants to determine whether applicants' skills fit the duties of the jobs they hope to fill. All of these interviewers (reporters, doctors, employers) are collecting information for particular purposes. Survey interviewers also collect information for particular purposes, purposes that are determined by the research questions posed during the design of the survey projects of which they are a part. As will become clear through the discussion in this book, however, the survey interviewer's task is different from that of other types of interviewers.

The in-person mode of survey administration has advantages and disadvantages when compared with self-administered and telephone-administered surveys. In-person interviews can be used in a variety of settings to gather data about a multitude of topics.

Who Participates in the Interview?

An interview usually involves two people: the **interviewer,** who asks prepared questions, and the **respondent,** who answers them. Interviews are also sometimes done "by proxy"—that is, someone other than the chosen respondent answers questions on behalf of the chosen respondent. Survey researchers sometimes use proxy respondents when their desired respondents cannot participate directly—for example, when the preferred respondents are very young children, persons with memory impairment (such as Alzheimer's patients), or deceased persons. Generally, however, a survey interview is a structured conversation between an interviewer and a respondent who has been selected through a predetermined sampling method. The respondent is chosen based on his or her being a member of a population of interest, often called the *target population.*

As noted above, the task with which survey interviewers are charged is somewhat different from that of other kinds of interviewers. Journalists, doctors, employers, and many others who participate in interview conversations do so with little restriction. They are allowed to interject comments, make educated judgments, and prompt respondents for further information according to their own instincts and skills. These interviewers are often also the "analysts" of the data they gather. The reporter writes his or her own article, the doctor makes a direct diagnosis, and the employer makes a personal judgment as to whether the applicant is right for the job. Researchers who conduct "qualitative" interviews personally may also conduct analyses of their own findings.

Most surveys, however, are conducted using **quantitative methods**—that is, methods that permit the measurement of findings using statistical methods. Interviewers working on quantitative surveys usually have nothing to do with the analysis of the data they gather. Especially in large-scale quantitative surveys, which may have hundreds of respondents, the surveyors (often with the help of analytic experts) perform the analysis of data, which involves complex statistical procedures. (In this book, the term *surveyors* is used to refer to the persons who pose the research questions, design the larger investigations within which surveys are done, and evaluate the meaning of the findings. These individuals, who are sometimes also called *investigators* or *researchers,* seldom conduct the interviews for the quantitative surveys in which they are involved.) It is the survey interviewer's job to uphold the necessary standardization in administering the questionnaire so as to make sure that the respondents' answers are valid and comparable at the analysis stage.

Standardization of administration means that every respondent is asked the same questions in the same way, with as little outside influence as possible. This means that interviewers must *not* participate substantively in conversation with respondents. Interviewers must understand that they are facilitators of data collection, and that they need to keep their own opinions out of their interviews. They need to read all questions as they are written in the questionnaire, keeping a neutral tone of voice. On the other hand, if interviewers behave like robots, respondents are likely to be put off, and this can affect their responses; they may become irritated and begin answering without thinking just to get through the interview, or they may refuse to answer at all. Interviewers must be able to maintain rapport with respondents without influencing their responses.

Thus the interviewer has the difficult dual task of keeping the interview at a conversational level while guiding the respondent along a prescribed path of questions and predetermined response alternatives. The negative effects that the interviewer may have on how the respondent answers questions are called **interviewer effects.** In-person interviewing is especially vulnerable to interviewer effects because the respondent is exposed not only to the interviewer's tone of voice (as he or she would be in a telephone interview) but also to visual cues such as race, age, body language, and facial expressions. All of these cues can inadvertently lead the respondent to answer questions in ways that reflect his or her attitude toward the interviewer rather than his or her responses to the questions per se.

What Does an Interview Consist Of?

The primary "what" of a survey interview is the **questionnaire**, also called the *survey instrument* or *survey tool.* Interview questionnaires are different from self-administered questionnaires in that the respondent does not see the questions. The interviewer reads the questions from the paper questionnaire or from a computer screen and records the answers. In addition to the questions, the questionnaire contains the script for the interviewer's part of the conversation. The path the interviewer is to take in moving through the questionnaire is clearly defined, as are the responses the interviewer is to offer to foreseeable questions or comments from the respondent. The questionnaire specifies standardized language that the interviewer must use for probing and prompting respondents who are confused or who give incomplete answers. The questionnaire also includes the script for the interviewer's introductory statements and closing remarks, as well as instructions for how the interviewer is to record the respondents' answers.

The questionnaire is constructed around content determined by the survey objectives. The format should create a flowing conversation. The interview process generally involves four tasks for the interviewer: making the introductory statement, screening for eligibility, obtaining informed consent, and asking the questions (which includes making the prescribed transition statements—scripted statements that introduce and separate different sections of the survey). In quantitative surveys, the questions usually come with predetermined response options, and respondents are asked to choose from finite lists of possible answers. Occasionally, open-ended questions (questions for which no preset response lists are offered) are included, however; for these, the interviewer must record respondents' answers verbatim.

Quantitative interviews are often completed by the paper-and-pencil interviewing (PAPI) method; the interviewer reads the questions from a paper questionnaire and records the respondent's answers directly onto the same document or onto a separate coding sheet. Special scannable coding sheets are developed for some survey projects, so that project staff members can scan respondents' answers directly into a computer for analysis without the step of key typing the responses the interviewer marked.

Interviewers sometimes administer quantitative surveys using **computer-assisted personal interviewing (CAPI)**. In this method, the interviewer reads the questions to the respondent from a computer screen rather than from a paper questionnaire and enters the respondent's answers directly into the computer via the keyboard. Programmers use specialized software to create questionnaires of this kind, which have some advantages over paper-and-pencil questionnaires. For example, in a CAPI survey, the computer automatically displays the next appropriate question, so that the interviewer does not have to follow any possibly confusing **skip patterns.** Questions meant only for women are automatically omitted, for example, if the respondent's gender is entered as male. CAPI programs can also automatically scan for inconsistent answers, thereby helping interviewers to catch data entry errors. Mathematical calculations can also be carried out within CAPI programs.

CAPI should not be confused with CATI (computer-assisted telephone interviewing) or CASI (computer-assisted self-interviewing). CAPI is conducted in person by live interviewers, often using portable computers. In contrast, CATI is conducted over the telephone by live interviewers using computerized survey instruments. CASI does not involve interviewers at all; rather, the respondents interact with computers directly.

When Is the In-Person Interview Mode Used?

When designing a survey, the surveyor must confront the decision of how it will be administered. Will the survey use interviewers (and, if so, will they interview in person or over the telephone), or will it involve a mailed, handed-out, or computerized questionnaire that respondents can fill out on their own? Surveyors often choose the in-person interview mode when they need to ask complex questions and/or the lists of response choices are long or may be confusing. This is because the physical presence of an interviewer often enhances interviewer-respondent rapport; it also allows for observation of nonverbal cues that may indicate confusion or hesitation on the part of the respondent.

In addition, interviewers can present respondents with visual aids during in-person interviews, making it easy for respondents to consider all of the response options. In telephone interviews, respondents have to keep all of the response options in memory, and in self-administered surveys, they might just skip difficult questions, or even abandon the questionnaire before finishing. In-person interviewing also tends to work best for long interviews, again because of the level of interviewer-respondent rapport that is possible when the two people are physically together. Certain populations are more easily interviewed in person, such as older people, who may have trouble hearing over the phone, and homeless people, who have no addresses (and so can't receive mail surveys) and no telephones (and so are not candidates for telephone-administered interviews).

However, in-person interviews are more vulnerable than telephone interviews to interviewer effects, and they tend to be more expensive than other types of surveys. If a survey requires respondents to travel to a study site for in-person interviews, or if interviewers must travel to respondents' homes or workplaces, the costs of transportation and extra interviewer time can be considerable. In-person interviews that can be done with many respondents in the same location (say, by intercepting people as they leave a particular store in a shopping mall) are less expensive. An important issue that the surveyor needs to consider in deciding whether to use this mode of administration is whether interviews can be conducted with a large enough sample. If the survey project is going to run out of money before enough people have been interviewed to answer the research questions, the surveyor should consider a less expensive mode. Surveyors need to weigh the advantages against the disadvantages in deciding whether the in-person mode is best for particular surveys.

Where Are In-Person Interviews Conducted?

In-person interviews can be conducted just about anywhere people can meet. The topic of the survey and issues of accessibility to the target population will influence the choice of locale. When an interview is to be done as part of a large health study that also involves medical examinations, collection of blood samples, or X rays, participants may be invited to a research site, perhaps at a clinic. The interview can be conducted privately, either on paper or on a computer, in a small office. Opinion polls are often conducted by interviewers who go door-to-door in preselected neighborhoods. Marketing research interviews may be done by interviewers who stand outside the doors of department stores in shopping malls. Interviewers might approach swimmers at a beach to conduct a survey to assess levels of exposure to water pollutants. Children may be called from their classrooms and interviewed in the school's cafeteria for a study of children's reactions to high-stakes testing. The possibilities are endless. For some studies, interviewers make themselves mobile by carrying paper questionnaires on clipboards; others carry laptop computers into the field.

Why Are In-Person Interviews Done?

Surveyors elect to use in-person interviews in their survey studies because, under the right circumstances, such interviews offer many advantages for valid (that is, accurate and precise) data collection. Compared with telephone-administered interviews, in-person interviews have the advantage that the interviewer can see how a respondent is reacting and can show the respondent items that help clarify questions and response options. Compared with self-administered surveys, both in-person and telephone interviews benefit from the interviewer's role in enhancing respondent participation by guiding questioning, answering the respondent's questions, and clarifying the meanings of responses.

Also, in interview surveys, the surveyor has control over the response pattern, because the interviewer determines the sequence of the questions; in a self-administered survey, respondents can answer the questions in any order (except in most surveys administered on computers). In addition, in self-administered surveys, persons other than the intended respondents can fill out questionnaires without the surveyor's knowledge. Another advantage of interviewing in general is that it allows the surveyor some control over the sample. Interviewers can often motivate reluctant respondents to go through with interviews, whereas mailed or handed-out surveys can end up in the garbage can. This limits the representativeness of the sample, because those who throw away the survey may differ in important characteristics from those who take the trouble to fill it out.

After the questions of who, what, when, where and why, the question that logically follows is "How?" The above overview of the five Ws of in-person survey interviewing is intended to provide some context for the discussion in the following chapters about *how* interviews are conducted: How does the surveyor identify and access the population? How do project staff members construct the questionnaire? How does the interviewer conduct the questioning? How does the interviewer use technological aids? How do supervisors hire, train, and supervise interviewers? How do project staff members manage interview data once completed surveys begin coming in from the field? How do surveyors and interviewers address cultural differences and language barriers?

Most surveys are done using quantitative methods, and most of the chapters in this volume describe how in-person interviews are conducted for quantitative investigations. There is another interview approach, however: the qualitative interview. Qualitative interviews take a number of forms, and studies that use qualitative interviews have goals and analysis procedures that are different from those of quantitative investigations. Qualitative studies usually have research questions that require *description* of how phenomena are experienced rather than measurement of aspects of experience. Qualitative methods are less concerned with standardization, and the focus is usually on eliciting great amounts of detail from a few respondents. Qualitative interviews have an important place as tools for information gathering and can be used in conjunction with quantitative surveys. Because the methods used in qualitative interviewing are different from those used in quantitative interviews, they are discussed separately, in Chapter 8.

2 How to Operationalize the Survey Design

The survey design (the environmental arrangement within which the survey is done) is usually set forth in a funding proposal or protocol that precedes implementation of the project. The surveyor poses the research questions and sets the survey objectives, and then, with the questions and objectives in mind, decides the characteristics required of respondents, how large the sample must be, how respondents will be identified, and what survey mode will be used. If the surveyor chooses the mode of in-person interviewing, he or she must also anticipate when and where respondents will be interviewed and what information will be sought in the interviews. (For a thorough discussion of survey design, see **How to Design Survey Studies**, Volume 6 in this series.)

The surveyor must then develop an administrative plan that lays out how the survey design will be operationalized—that is, how it will be put into action in the real world, and according to what timeline. The surveyor must create a budget by estimating all the costs of implementing the survey, such as space rental, payment of staff and consultants, costs of purchase or rental of equipment, and costs of storage. Once funding is secured for the project, either from within an organization or from an outside agency such as a foundation or government institute, the work of "setting up shop" for the survey can begin.

In the start-up phase of a project, the survey team must usually answer three questions:

1. What combination of staff and resources will yield the highest-quality (most valid and reliable) survey data?

2. What can we reasonably accomplish within the necessary time line?

3. What can we actually afford?

Finding a balance among the answers to these questions will guide the survey logistics in the following core areas:

- Identification and location of enough eligible subjects
- Interview construction
- Interview administration
- Data tracking
- Data preparation and storage
- Data analysis
- Dissemination of findings

It can be difficult for surveyors to anticipate just how many people will need to be hired for certain tasks, how many computers will need to be purchased, how many hours of consultant time might be needed, and how much space will be needed to house employees, equipment, and data. They may be able to make some estimates by doing some pretesting of the survey instrument. For example, they can test a draft of the interview with a few real subjects in the expected setting for the real interviews. This may help the surveyors to anticipate how many respondents a single interviewer can interview in one day, and from this number they can estimate how many interviewers will be needed to get the desired total number of interviews in the available time. However, surveyors need to be flexible and willing to respond to circumstances as the survey develops over time. Many factors that can affect a survey simply cannot be anticipated well. Plans will have to be made and changed as the project unfolds.

Identification and Location of Enough Eligible Subjects

It is important that project personnel be true to the survey design in approaching the task of actually finding people to interview. How the population is to be sampled (whether a convenience or probability sample; see **How to Sample in Surveys**, Volume 7 in this series) and the number of interviews needed to answer the research questions to a degree of statistical certainty (the sample size) will influence decisions about how many recruiters and interviewers should be hired and how their job descriptions should be written. Recruiters (personnel who find possible subjects, screen them for eligibility, and ultimately recruit them to participate in the survey) must be trained to follow the sampling strategy outlined in the survey protocol. In some surveys, interviewers perform both recruiting and interviewing tasks, whereas in others, recruiters do only participant identification and screening and then pass eligible and willing respondents along to interviewers.

Systematic procedures need to be put in place for screening, selecting, and recruiting possible respondents. In addition, a filing system needs to be developed that will allow project personnel to look up completed interviews for error correction and to avoid duplication of work.

Interview Construction

The survey topic and objectives determine the content of the questionnaire. For in-person interviews, the designers of the questionnaire develop interviewer instructions as well as conventions for separating instructions from what the interviewer is to read to the respondent (see Chapter 6). The surveyor may prepare the questionnaire personally or solicit expertise from paid consultants or colleagues. If the survey is to be administered by computer, the surveyor may enlist the help of a programmer familiar with CAPI software to translate the paper questionnaire into an electronic version. The surveyor needs to plan for the time and interview staff required to pretest drafts of the survey until it is deemed ready to be put into the field.

Interview Administration

Surveyors must hire interviewers and provide them with training in the techniques of standardized interviewing. Personnel must also be hired to supervise the interviewers. Supervisors will develop mechanisms to ensure that all recruiters and interviewers follow procedures in the same way. These might take the form of weekly meetings or conference calls, or perhaps supervisors will attend interviews at random.

The surveyor may consult with colleagues to work out fieldwork strategies. Will interviews be conducted in subjects' homes, workplaces, or other designated meeting places? Will an interview center be set up where subjects are asked to come in? If so, will they be reimbursed for transportation costs? What data quality checks will be implemented? How will supervisors monitor response rates, refusal rates, interviewer error, and interviewer and recruiter support needs?

Will incentive payments or gifts be offered to subjects as a gesture of thanks for participating? If interviews are done by CAPI, how many portable computers must be purchased for home interviews? Or how many desktop computers are needed for the interviewing center? How will interviewers transport the things they need to take into the field? How much will they be reimbursed for mileage if they need to use their own vehicles to travel to meet with respondents?

Data Tracking

Lost data are a surveyor's worst nightmare. A great deal of effort and cost is invested in every interview that is done. It is important to be sure that every interview makes it from the point of data collection to the point of data analysis. Project staff must develop logs, face sheets, and data backup mechanisms so that missing interviews can be identified and looked for. When interviews are done in large volume and/or equipment and supplies are carted from the field to the survey office and back to the field, things *can and will* get lost.

Every interview should be assigned several identifiers. Because confidentiality agreements (see Chapter 5) usually prohibit use of respondents' names to identify specific interviews, surveyors often assign a study number to each respondent. If necessary, the identity of a given person can be cross-referenced to the ID number, as in a situation where a person's answers before and after exposure to a stimulus (say, watching a commercial) need to be compared.

Project staff should keep a confidential log that cross-references respondents' names, ID numbers, and other identifying information (e.g., gender, birth date, recruitment location, date of study entry) in a secure location to which only study personnel have access. Because ID numbers can be recorded incorrectly, it is advisable for the surveyor to collect at least one or two other identifiers in the interview itself, such as gender, birth date, and date of interview. Then, if an ID number is entered incorrectly, a staff member can look up a log entry based on birth date and find the correct ID.

To track whether all interviews done are actually received for data entry, the surveyor should institute a separate paper trail, either by logging every interview done or by preparing a face sheet that summarizes the basic details of the interview. The log or face sheet should reflect the ID number of the particular interview, the date of the interview, the name of the interviewer, and any particularly important outcomes of the interview that the surveyor would most want to know should the interview be lost in its entirety. Interviewers keep a log or turn in face sheets separately from the interviews themselves, and a manager or programmer matches the log or face sheet entries to the paper or CAPI interviews received to see if anything is missing. This should be done on an ongoing and frequent basis, because the more recently something has been misplaced, the more likely it is the interviewer will be able to retrieve it.

Another concern is that data could be destroyed inadvertently. Everyone has had the experience of losing work to a computer malfunction, and paper interviews can be lost in a variety of ways, including flooding or fire in a storage area. The surveyor should have interviewers make backup copies (whether photocopies or electronic backup files) of all interviews before forwarding them to the project for further processing. The backups should be kept in a location separate from the original interviews; that is, paper copies and originals should be in different rooms, offices, or storage lockers, and electronic copies should not be stored on the same computer as the originals.

Data Preparation and Storage

Once the interviews have been administered, editors and programmers process and store the data for analysis. The first step is the **editing** of the completed interviews. For paper interviews, this usually means that a supervisor or an interviewer other than the one who conducted the interview goes through each questionnaire to look for inconsistent answers and obvious errors in recording of information. In the case of CAPI interviews, many such errors are impossible to make, because the program guides the interviewer through the questioning. Still, an interviewer can enter responses incorrectly on the keyboard, and sometimes interviewers may misinterpret respondents' intentions. Interviewers are trained to record verbatim, as text notes in the questionnaire, any clarifying remarks a respondent makes. Editors of both paper and CAPI interviews compare these recorded comments to the answer choices marked by the interviewers to make sure the coding seems to be correct. If there is doubt, the editor might contact the interviewer or the respondent for clarification, or the surveyor may make an executive decision about how the item should be coded. Any necessary corrections should be made before the interview data are processed further.

Survey data usually cannot be analyzed directly from the paper or computerized questionnaires on which they are collected. The programmer must translate the data for accessibility to a computer software program (usually a statistical program such as SAS or SPSS) that can combine answers across interviews in order to calculate statistics. For a CAPI survey, a programmer can write a program that will make the CAPI data "comprehensible" to the statistical program. If the data are on paper, they need to be converted into an electronic form, either through scanning of completed "bubble" response sheets or through keyboard entry. **Data entry** personnel can be hired and trained, or the interviews can be delivered to an independent company for data entry and returned to the study in electronic form on disk or tape.

Once the data are in a form the statistical program can read, the programmer will search for missing item-level data and run checks for out-of-range answers (answers that do not correspond to any response options or that are impossible based on previous answers). The programmer carries out a process called *data cleaning,* preferably on an ongoing basis. When answers are missing or seem to be incorrect, the supervisor may contact the interviewer and sometimes the respondent in an effort to replace the incorrect data with correct information. Once the data are considered to be as "clean" as possible, the programmer stores multiple copies of the data set on different computers or on backup disks and tapes kept in a different location. As interviewers complete more interviews over time, the programmer cleans the data and adds the new data to the existing data set. The cumulative cleaned data are eventually used for analyses.

Data Analysis

Although the surveyor may request that preliminary analyses be carried out before the entire sample has been interviewed, the primary analyses will be done when all of the data are in. It is important, however, that the surveyor be aware of the complexity of the anticipated analyses at the time of survey setup, so that he or she can seek the proper level of advice from statistical collaborators and consultants and can acquire the required statistical packages and other software at the right time. Alternatively, the surveyor may plan to farm out the analyses (for a fee) to appropriate experts who have the required electronic capabilities. Communication is extremely important at this stage of the survey study: The surveyor must make sure that the analyses that are performed correctly address the original research questions and that those who report the data in publications and/or use the data to make decisions understand what the findings drawn from the analyses mean.

Dissemination of Findings

Although issues of dissemination do not usually come up until much of the survey work per se is finished, the surveyor should anticipate what form the dissemination will take and who will be responsible for producing the products. Many survey projects result in scholarly journal articles that disseminate findings to the surveyor's colleagues in the field. Other forms of dissemination might be the production of teaching tools based on survey findings and talks given at conferences. A company may disseminate survey findings internally, via reports or meetings, to help with decision making about product development or advertising. The surveyor should try to be clear about the long-term goals of the project during the setup phase, so that adequate resources can be reserved for staff time to accomplish these important final steps.

The process of "setting up shop" to conduct a survey requires attention to a great many factors if it is to be done efficiently and cost-effectively. The need for communication at every step cannot be overemphasized. Mechanisms for linking all members of the team in carrying out decisions and understanding goals are crucial. Communication through e-mail, conference calls, and regular meetings of key staff members and documentation in the form of written notes and minutes are essential to the smooth flow of a project. Some surveyors also find it very helpful to create a project identity by choosing a logo for use on stationery and other materials related to the project. Depending on the scope and nature of the survey, a project Web site might also be developed, funds permitting.

The following checklist summarizes the elements a surveyor should consider during setup of a project, including design, timeline, and funding constraints. Certainly, many aspects of the start-up of a project will be carried out simultaneously. Among the highest-priority tasks in the early going is, of course, construction of the survey itself; that is the subject of Chapter 3.

Project Setup Checklist

✓ Project identity/logo/Web site development

✓ Office space and storage needs

✓ Staffing needs: project coordinator, recruiters, interviewers, programmer, statistician, psychometrician, consultants

✓ Plan for survey content and assembly

✓ Plan for recruiter and interviewer training

✓ Plan for subject identification, screening, and recruitment

✓ Choice of survey administration site (homes, office, or other)

✓ Equipment needs (computers, scanner, printer, and so on)

✓ Transportation needs (for interviewers and/or respondents)

✓ Tracking methods (ID numbering, logs, face sheets, data backup)

✓ Supervisory routines (checks of sampling procedures, response rate, validation)

✓ Plan for interview editing and data cleaning

✓ Plan for data entry considerations (if paper interviews)

✓ Plan for analysis

✓ Plan for dissemination of findings

✓ Confidentiality considerations

✓ Offer of participant incentives

3 How to Design an Interview for In-Person Administration

An extensive literature is available on the art and science of questionnaire construction. Much of the accumulated wisdom on this topic applies generically to all types of surveys, not just to those administered by in-person interview. This chapter focuses on some very general guidelines for questionnaire construction, highlighting a few points that apply particularly to in-person interviewing. For additional details, especially on special question-writing techniques, see **How to Design Survey Studies** (Volume 6 in this series) as well as the works listed in the "Suggested Readings" section at the end of this book. Although such techniques are useful for all types of surveys, some apply more specifically to telephone interviewing and are not covered here.

Interview Questions

Designing questions for interviews is a complex process that involves many considerations. The basic task is twofold: Write the questions and organize them into a coherent document—the questionnaire. The goals of question *writing* are to capture content relevant to the survey objectives in language that is meaningful to the target group and with a presentation style that maximizes the likelihood of obtaining valid responses. The goals of questionnaire *organization* are to create smooth conversational flow for both the respondent and the interviewer and to provide structure for interview programming (if the survey is to be administered by computer) and data entry.

CONTENT

The primary purpose of the questions is to meet the objectives of the survey. To decide on the content of survey questions, the surveyor must operationalize the problems the survey is expected to address. The surveyor can do this by listing topic areas, or variables, that must be covered in an interview and/or ideas about the relationships among variables. Once these variables have been defined, the surveyor can make decisions about how they will be measured. The basic steps are listed in the following checklist.

Checklist for Determining Question Content

✓ List the survey objectives.

✓ Conceptualize the components of each objective by listing relevant topics.

✓ Frame questions for each topic.

Example 3.1 illustrates how a surveyor might go about capturing the survey objectives in the questions. Surveyors may write the questions for their surveys entirely from scratch, or they may borrow measures from previously validated surveys. For example, the surveyor in Example 3.1 could conceptualize that depression is a common factor contributing to low quality of life among women in the target population. Women who are very depressed may find it difficult to make use of services and express dissatisfaction with the program or, on the other hand, may find that their depression symptoms improve as a result of participation. The surveyor could find a validated depression scale in the literature and use it in the survey to identify respondents who may suffer from depressive symptoms. If program participants are surveyed twice, once before and once after participation in the program, the surveyor could compare depression scores and satisfaction outcomes.

EXAMPLE 3.1
Operationalizing the Survey Problem

A survey has the following objective: to assess satisfaction among participants of a perinatal outreach program for underserved women in Los Angeles County.

The surveyor first operationalizes satisfaction by listing relevant topics:

1. Levels of satisfaction with specific program services

2. Reasons for dissatisfaction with program services

3. Perceived impact of program services on quality of life

4. Suggestions for program improvement

Example 3.1 continued

The surveyor then develops the questions to measure satisfaction:

1. The first question set asks about satisfaction with each program service (referrals to prenatal care, transportation to prenatal visits, baby-sitting during prenatal visits, and housing assistance). The respondent is asked whether she needed each service and, if so, whether the service was provided by the program. If her response is yes, she is asked how satisfied she was with the service, using a scale ranging from *extremely satisfied* to *extremely dissatisfied.*

2. The next set of questions refers the respondent back to every service with which she said she was dissatisfied. She is then asked why she was dissatisfied. No response options are offered because the surveyor does not want to influence what might be said. Possible responses are anticipated, however, and are listed for easy checkoff by the interviewer. Space for unanticipated responses is also provided.

3. Because the surveyor conceptualizes satisfaction to include a sense that quality of life has been improved by program participation, a third set of questions asks whether program participation improved the respondent's quality of life. For purposes of this survey, *quality of life* is defined as lowered daily stress level, improved sense of overall well-being, improved sense of personal health, and

Example 3.1 continued

increased expectation of a healthy delivery. The respondent is asked to what degree program participation improved her quality of life in each area (on a scale ranging from *very much* to *not at all*).

4. The questionnaire ends with an open-ended question (that is, a question for which no possible answers are provided for the respondent to choose from) asking for suggestions for program improvement.

WORDING

Specific guidelines for formulating survey objectives and determining variables of interest, together with the mechanics of question wording, question types, formatting, and use of scales, are described in **How to Ask Survey Questions** (Volume 2 in this series). The following checklist offers a few general guidelines and notes some common errors; each of the items in the checklist is discussed briefly below.

General Checklist for Question Wording

✓ Use language that is comprehensible to the target population.

✓ Keep the wording neutral.

✓ Ask about one concept or issue per question.

✓ Include enough information so that respondents can give meaningful answers (that is, so that most respondents don't say, "I don't know").

✓ Provide response options that are exhaustive and mutually exclusive.

Language Relevant to the Population

When writing the questions described in Example 3.1, the surveyor must take into account the characteristics, such as age and educational background, of the respondents. The example notes that the respondents are to be asked whether program participation improved their overall sense of well-being. The women in the target group may have limited formal education and may not speak fluent English. For this population, a question such as "How did participation in this program affect your overall sense of well-being?" might be confusing, requiring prompting instructions for the surveyor's meaning of the concept of "well-being." Because the surveyor is interested in a simple understanding of whether women "feel better" than they did before program participation, a simpler approach may be more meaningful: "Since you started participating in this program, have you been feeling better, the same, or worse in your everyday life?" Putting the question into more direct language may improve understanding of the surveyor's intent and improve rapport between interviewer and respondent.

Neutrality

An interview question should not imply that any particular answer is preferred over others. This implication can occur when inflammatory words are used, or when there is emotional content in the wording. A question like "Would you support legislation that gives disadvantaged kids a fighting chance?" implies that the surveyor may be emotionally invested in such legislation—that is, there is a suggestion of something to "fight" for. It also doesn't really tell the respondent what the legislation is about. A better question might be "Would you support legislation that provides after-school sports programs for children from low-income families?" This language provides more detail and is less emotional. Questions that imply a preferred response are sometimes called **loaded questions.**

One Concept

Combining more than one concept or issue in a single question is a common mistake made by surveyors. Such **double-barreled questions** confuse the respondent, and the surveyor ultimately does not know which part of these questions the respondent actually answered. A question like "What is your preferred mode of transportation when it's raining or snowing?" might seem an appropriate way to ask how respondents like to travel in bad weather, but it assumes that respondents prefer the same mode of transportation under two different weather conditions. It does not allow for the possibility, for instance, that some respondents might prefer to take the bus when it's raining, but want to drive their own cars with snow chains on snowy days. It is better to ask about each condition in a separate question.

Too Many "I Don't Knows"

It is usually best to keep questions as simple as possible, but sometimes respondents will not know enough about a topic to give an opinion if the question contains too few details. If nearly everyone answers "I don't know" to a particular question, the surveyor ends up with useless data for that question. For example, "How do you feel about the recent changes in the city buses?" is a vague question that assumes respondents will know which changes are being referred to. Unsure of the intent of the question, respondents are likely to say, "I don't know," even if they did notice the change the surveyor has in mind. "How do you feel about the new seats in the city's recently renovated buses?" is more specific and meaningful.

Exhaustive and Exclusive Response Options

It is easy to overlook the importance of clear **response options.** The response options are part of every survey question (except those that are open-ended) and must be as carefully written as the question itself. There must be enough choices to cover all or most possible answers, and response choices must not overlap, or respondents will not know how to choose the best answer and the surveyor will have unclear results. Consider this question: "How would you describe the weather in your neighborhood last week? Sunny, cloudy, or rainy?" The response options for this question are neither exhaustive nor exclusive. It could have been snowing most of the week or it could have been cloudy *and* rainy all week. It is also important that choices do not overlap. It is sometimes easy to miss that certain answers could fall into two of the offered response categories. For example, for the question "What is your age?" some surveyors might make the mistake of offering these options: younger than 20, 20-30, 30-40, 40-50, older than 50. Respondents who happen to be exactly 20, 30, or 40 years old would fall into two of the offered categories. Better categories might be as follows: younger than 20, 20-29, 30-39, 40-49, 50 or older.

Following are some additional guidelines for surveyors concerning the wording of questions.

Visual Aids

One of the main advantages that in-person interviewing has over other modes of survey administration is the opportunity to use visual aids. Whereas other types of surveys must rely heavily on question-writing techniques to help respondents deal with difficult question styles (such as questions requiring long lists of response choices), in-person interviews often use visual aids to assist the respondent. Such aids are helpful when respondents are faced with complex or long questions and response lists or with questions requiring rankings, recall, or visual estimates.

COMPLEX OR LONG QUESTIONS AND RESPONSE LISTS

Whenever possible, it is best to keep questions and response lists short and simple. However, if a complex question is simplified too much, it may generate a large number of "no opinion" responses because respondents don't have enough information to formulate opinions. Before asking a complex question, the surveyor may need to give the respondent detailed background information. This information can be printed on a card, so that the interviewer can hand the card to the respondent and ask the respondent to read along on the card as the interviewer reads the same information aloud from the questionnaire.

When response choices are complicated or very numerous, respondents can find it difficult to remember the first choice by the time the last one is read. Sometimes limiting response categories can be a problem for the surveyor, because a shorter list of options may not provide enough detail for the data to be meaningful. Example 3.2 illustrates how visual aids, in the form of flash cards containing the same lists of response options the interviewer sees on the questionnaire, can help respondents to answer some questions.

EXAMPLE 3.2
Visual Aids for Complex Responses and Long Lists of Responses

Complex Response Options

QUESTION
Regarding physical activity, compared to others of your age and sex, when you were (read age group below), were you (read choices)?

Example 3.2 continued

(Show Flash Card H)

	Much Less Active	Less Active	Average	More Active	Much More Active
Teens and early 20s	1	2	3	4	5
Late 20s and 30s	1	2	3	4	5
40s	1	2	3	4	5
50s	1	2	3	4	5
60s	1	2	3	4	5
70s	1	2	3	4	5

Comment: Flash Card H allows the respondent to study the complex list of response options to determine his or her answer for each relevant age. With the flash card as an aid, the respondent is unlikely to forget any of the choices offered.

FLASH CARD H

	MUCH LESS ACTIVE	LESS ACTIVE	AVERAGE	MORE ACTIVE	MUCH MORE ACTIVE
TEENS AND EARLY 20s	1	2	3	4	5
LATE 20s AND 30s	1	2	3	4	5
40s	1	2	3	4	5
50s	1	2	3	4	5
60s	1	2	3	4	5
70s	1	2	3	4	5

SOURCE: Kaiser/UCLA Sigmoid Study.

Example 3.2 continued

Long List of Complex Responses

QUESTION   What is your natural adult hair color?

(Show Flash Card I)

Bright red	1
Red	2
Light blonde	3
Blonde (whole life)	4
Light brown (blonde as child)	5
Light brown (whole life)	6
Medium brown	7
Auburn (dark red-brown)	8
Dark brown/black	9
Jet black	10

Comment: This list of response options not only involves complexity (different shades of hair color at different times of life), it is also rather long. The respondent would likely find this list very difficult to retain in memory if it were just spoken out loud, but using the flash card, the respondent can review the choices as needed in responding to the question.

FLASH CARD I

BRIGHT RED	**LIGHT BROWN (WHOLE LIFE)**
RED	**MEDIUM BROWN**
LIGHT BLONDE	**AUBURN (DARK RED-BROWN)**
BLONDE (WHOLE LIFE)	**DARK BROWN/BLACK**
LIGHT BROWN (BLONDE AS CHILD)	**JET BLACK**

SOURCE: Kaiser UCLA Sigmoid Study.

RANKING

Visual aids are also useful for questions that require the respondent to rank items (that is, put items in order according to some criterion—for example, most important to least important). In the in-person interview, ranking is easily accomplished: The interviewer hands the respondent a list of the items to be ranked or a set of cards with one item on each, which the respondent can simply sort into rank order.

EXAMPLE 3.3
Visual Aid for Listing
Response Options for Priority Choice

QUESTION
Now, thinking about the chance of property damage, injuries, public health problems, and the loss of life, please rank the following hazards in order from most to least threatening to your community today.

HAND CARD TO RESPONDENT.
RECORD RANK ORDER IN RIGHT COLUMN.

Hazard	Ranking
Tornadoes	
Floods	
Earthquakes	
Water pollution	
Nuclear/radiation accident	
Hazardous chemical spill	
Don't know	

Example 3.3 continued

RESPONSE CARD

HAZARDS

Tornadoes

Floods

Earthquakes

Water Pollution

Nuclear/Radiation Accident

Hazardous Chemical Spill

Comment: Using this visual aid, the respondent simply names the responses in the order he or she considers to be most to least threatening. The interviewer records the rankings in the appropriate boxes on the interview form or computer screen; the first hazard named is ranked 1, the second 2, and so on.

RECALL TECHNIQUES

Surveyors use special techniques to enhance response accuracy when designing questions that require respondents to recall events. The problem of *omission,* or forgetting an event entirely, can be addressed using a form of aided recall. Visual aids are one option. For example, a surveyor can stimulate recall by presenting a list of events or behaviors and asking if the respondent has taken part in them. Instead of asking the open-ended question "What leisure activities have you participated in during the past year?" the surveyor provides a list of activities and asks the respondent to choose from the list all that apply. For telephone interviews, such lists must be short (although several sets can be presented separately), but in-person interviewers can simply hand the lists to respondents for review, to make sure nothing is omitted.

Another problem of recall questions, *telescoping,* or the tendency to report events as having taken place more recently than they actually did, can be lessened if respondents can verify their answers with records. For example, a respondent might be encouraged to consult his or her weekly planner to verify the actual date of the last homeowner's association meeting attended. During the in-person interview, the interviewer can wait while respondents locate any documents they need to verify their answers.

Another approach to aiding recall is to use landmark events as reference points. For example, a respondent could be asked if a behavior occurred before or after the last election. Holidays and celebrations, major disasters, noteworthy international events such as the Olympic Games, and high-profile media publicity surrounding events like the O. J. Simpson trial are examples of landmark occurrences that can serve as adequate time referents because they are generally known to everyone. The in-person interviewer can show the respondent a calendar or timeline on which landmark events are marked to assist the respondent in reconstructing the timing of events.

VISUAL ESTIMATES

In addition to helping respondents cope with complex or long lists of response options, rankings, and questions requiring recall, visual aids can help respondents deal with scales that require estimations, as illustrated in Example 3.4.

EXAMPLE 3.4
Visual Aid for a Rating Scale
Requiring a Visual Estimate

QUESTION

I'm going to ask you how you feel about various government agencies and institutions. Please tell me how much you trust . . .

| NO | | | | | | | | | | COMPLETE |
| TRUST | | | | | | | | | | TRUST |

The president

| 0 | 1 | 2 | 3 | 4 | 5 | 6 | 7 | 8 | 9 | 10 |

VISUAL AID

RATING SCALE—TRUST										
NO										COMPLETE
TRUST										TRUST
0	1	2	3	4	5	6	7	8	9	10

Comment: Using this visual aid, the respondent can estimate the amount of trust he or she has in the president by looking at the scale and specifying a point that corresponds to that amount.

The uses and types of visual aids that can be used in in-person interviews are virtually limitless. Some of the more common ones (including those described above) are as follows:

- Lists of response options (if complex or numerous)

- Lists of items to aid recall

- Rating scales for questions requiring visual estimates

- Information summaries relevant to the respondent's forming opinions for a question or question sequence

- Lists of informative items to educate the respondent

- Lists from which the respondent makes priority choices

- Photographs (e.g., pictures of medications) to aid recall

- Cards containing one item each for ranking

- Calendars to aid recall of timing of events

- Maps to clarify geographic relationships

Surveyors may also develop many other kinds of visual aids. The design of such aids is part of the task of question writing. For survey modes that do not employ interviewers or in which interviews are done by telephone, surveyors must use question-writing techniques to overcome the limitations of not being able to use and explain visual aids. Some of the same question-writing techniques may be useful for in-person interviews, but they may be less necessary when surveyors can use visual aids (see the sources listed in the "Suggested Readings" section at the end of this book for more information on question-writing techniques).

The in-person interview mode has one other related advantage. When it comes to sensitive interview questions, such as those relating to sexuality, racial issues, or drug use, it can be difficult to know whether respondents feel comfortable enough with the interviewer and the survey's level of confidentiality to speak freely. In the in-person interview mode, the interviewer can do most of the interview orally, but hand certain questions to the respondent in an envelope for completion in private. The respondent can then seal the page with his or her answers in the envelope, which is not marked with a name or other identifier, other than perhaps a study ID number for later data entry by an anonymous data entry person. In this way, the advantages of the in-person interview are maintained for the bulk of the interview, and the answers to sensitive questions are less influenced by the respondent's need to provide **socially desirable responses** to an interviewer (that is, answers that the respondent thinks are generally acceptable or "politically correct" even though they may not reflect the respondent's actual views).

Writing questions and developing aids for their administration is one part of questionnaire construction. The next task is the organization of those questions.

Questionnaire Organization and Format

Once the questions and any visual aids have been developed, they must be organized into a questionnaire. *Organization* here refers not only to the order in which the questions are presented but also to the instructional guidelines for the interviewer and programmer or data entry person that hold all of the parts of the questionnaire together. The task of organizing the interview questions should be guided by two primary criteria: the "flow" of the questionnaire and potential question-order effects. In creating the transitions from question to question and from question group to question group, the surveyor needs to consider the expectations and tasks of the interviewer, the respondent, and the programmer or data entry person. To minimize the effect of question order on response patterns, the surveyor must give careful consideration to how respondents' exposure to one question might influence how they answer subsequent questions.

Following the guidelines below can help the surveyor to maintain the conversational flow of the interview while also providing clarity and logic for the respondent and the data entry person or programmer. Smooth question sequencing makes the tasks of both the respondent and the interviewer easier; disorganized interviewing increases error from inaccurate responses and results in lower response rates.

Guidelines for Questionnaire Flow

- Use a smooth conversational tone in all portions of the interview that are read to the respondent. This includes instructions, probes, and prompts.

- Set up the page so that interviewer instructions and programming or coding guidelines are clearly distinguishable from the portions to be read aloud to the respondent; you can accomplish this by using different capitalization styles and typefaces, and by employing graphics, such as instruction boxes. One of the best ways to distinguish instructions from questions is to use all capital letters for the instructions to interviewers. (Programming instructions are not visible on the screen in a CAPI survey, but they must be present on the paper draft to guide the programmer in setting up the interview using computer-assisted interviewing, or CAI, software.)

- Use written directions and arrows to guide the interviewer through the form. Even if the interviewer is to administer the questionnaire using a computer, it is advisable to have available paper versions of the questionnaire with clear instructions. Technology has been known to fail occasionally, requiring paper-and-pencil interviews to be done.

- Avoid organizing items in a way that requires the interviewer to page back and forth in the questionnaire. If the interviewer will need to refer to information given previously, repeat it.

The questionnaire items shown in Example 3.5 illustrate interviewer instructions that enhance flow. In this example, **transition statements** (statements that introduce and separate sections) appear in all capital letters, instructions to the interviewer are in italics, and skip patterns are marked with arrows followed by the numbers of the questions to which the interviewer should skip. These conventions apply only to this particular questionnaire; a questionnaire designed by another surveyor or for another purpose might use different conventions. Throughout any given questionnaire, however, the surveyor should adopt standardized conventions to keep the interviewer from getting lost on the page or reading something aloud that is not intended for the respondent to hear.

EXAMPLE 3.5
Instructions to Enhance Flow

1. FIRST, I'D LIKE TO START BY ASKING YOU SOME GENERAL QUESTIONS ABOUT YOURSLF.

   What is your date of birth?

   _____/_____/_____

   Month   Day   Year

   (*Compute current age here:* _____ *years;* *also code age on p. 27*)

Example 3.5 continued

2. What is your current marital status?

Married	1	
Widowed	2	→ SKIP TO Q4
Separated or divorced	3	→ SKIP TO Q4
Never married	4	→ SKIP TO Q4

3. Do you live with your wife/husband?

Yes	1	→ SKIP TO Q6
No	2	

4. Do you live alone?

Yes	1	→ SKIP TO Q6
No	2	

5. Do you live with other family members or with someone else?

*(Circle only one; if respondent lives with other family members, circle 1 even if respondent **also** lives with someone else.)*

With other family members	1
With someone else	2

6. NOW I WOULD LIKE TO LEARN MORE ABOUT MEMBERS OF YOUR FAMILY.

(Go to the SUPPLEMENT for the questions to use with this section.)

SOURCE: Kaiser/UCLA Sigmoid Study.

All of the anticipated answers in the questionnaire fragment in Example 3.5 already have codes assigned (e.g., in Question 2, married is coded 1, widowed is coded 2, and so on), making the task of recording responses very straightforward. The interviewer simply circles the number of the answer given. The data entry person then has no problem transferring responses to the database because they are already coded. In any cases where responses could be coded in a variety of ways (as for open-ended questions), standardized coding instructions to the interviewer should be printed on the form to make coding, and therefore data entry, as clear as possible.

When designing an interview to be administered by an interviewer using a computer, the surveyor needs to provide **computer-assisted interviewing (CAI)** instructions to the programmer throughout a preliminary paper version of the questionnaire, as shown in Example 3.6. In this example, coding and skipping instructions are in all capital letters for the interviewer. The same skipping instructions are given for the CAI programmer; these are set off in boxes so that they are easy for the programmer to see. The boxes and the skipping instructions to the interviewer do not appear on the screen once the questions have been programmed for CAPI. Thus there is less clutter on the screen than on the paper interview to confuse the interviewer, and skipping is automatically taken care of by the computer.

EXAMPLE 3.6
Programming Instructions for CAPI Interviews

EMPLOYMENT

H1. Now I'm going to ask some questions about your current employment situation. Are you . . . ?

[DO NOT PROBE BUT RECORD ALL THAT APPLY]

  1. now working
     (GO TO NEXT STATUS OR TO H2)

  2. temporarily laid off (SKIP TO H1c)

  3. unemployed and looking for work
     (SKIP TO H1b)

Example 3.6 continued

    4. disabled and unable to work (SKIP TO H1e)

    5. retired (GO TO H1a)

    6. a homemaker, or
       (GO TO NEXT STATUS OR TO H2)

    7. something else?
       (SPECIFY) _____
       (GO TO NEXT STATUS OR TO H2)

    8. DK

    9. REF

CAI: IF H1 = 5, DISPLAY H1a

H1a. In what month and year did you retire?

_ _ / _ _ _ _ MM/YYYY (GO TO NEXT STATUS OR TO H2)

DK   98   9998   (GO TO NEXT STATUS OR TO H2)
REF   99   9999   (GO TO NEXT STATUS OR TO H2)

CAI: IF H1 = 3, DISPLAY H1b

H1b. In what month and year did you become unemployed?

_ _ / _ _ _ _ MM/YYYY (GO TO NEXT STATUS OR TO H2)

DK   98   9998   (GO TO NEXT STATUS OR TO H2)
REF   99   9999   (GO TO NEXT STATUS OR TO H2)

CAI: IF H1 = 2, DISPLAY H1c

H1c. Do you expect to go back to this job?

    1. YES

    2. NO
       (GO TO NEXT STATUS OR TO H2)

Example 3.6 continued

    3. DK
        (GO TO NEXT STATUS OR TO H2)

    4. REF
        (GO TO NEXT STATUS OR TO H2)

CAI: IF H1 = 2, DISPLAY H1d

H1d. In what month and year did you last work on this job?

$\_\_/\_\_\_\_$ (GO TO NEXT STATUS OR TO H2)

DK   98   9998 (GO TO NEXT STATUS OR TO H2)
REF 99   9999 (GO TO NEXT STATUS OR TO H2)

CAI: IF H1 = 4, DISPLAY H1e

H1e. In what month and year did you become disabled?

$\_\_/\_\_\_\_$ (GO TO NEXT STATUS OR TO H2)

DK   98   9998 (GO TO NEXT STATUS OR TO H2)
REF 99   9999 (GO TO NEXT STATUS OR TO H2)

H2. Are you working for pay at the present time?
CAI: IF R IS WORKING NOW H1=1 CODE 1 AT H2 AND SKIP TO H3)

    1. YES
    5. NO   (SKIP TO H4)
    8. DK   (SKIP TO H4)
    9. REF   (SKIP TO H4)

SOURCE: Project IMPACT and Center for Health Studies, Group Health Cooperative.

Another type of programming instruction is the "fill" instruction. A nice feature of computer-assisted interviewing is that questions can be customized based on answers to previous questions. Example 3.7 shows an excerpt of a questionnaire with CAI programming instructions regarding two previous questions, Question B1, which asks the respondent's gender, and Question 2a, which asks if the respondent lives with a spouse. Combining this information, the computer program can determine whether the word *husband, wife,* or *partner* should be used (filled in) for Question B3. If the respondent's gender was filled in as male, the Question B3 that the interviewer will see on the computer screen and read to the respondent will automatically read, "Other than your wife, how many people do you live with?"

EXAMPLE 3.7
A Fill Instruction

CAI FILL PHRASE IN PARENTHESES: IF QB1 = 1 AND QB2a = 1, FILL "wife." IF QB1 = 2 AND QB2a = 1, FILL "husband." IF QB2 = 2, FILL "partner."

B3. Other than you and your (husband/wife/partner), how many people live with you?

_ _ PEOPLE   (IF 0, SKIP TO QB5, ELSE SKIP TO QB4)

98 DK   (SKIP TO QB5)
99 REF (SKIP TO QB5)

SOURCE: Project IMPACT and Center for Health Studies, Group Health Cooperative.

The programmer can also be instructed to program on-the-spot calculations based on a series of responses. Example 3.8 displays the instructions to the CAI programmer regarding a series of questions related to depression symptoms (not shown). The programmer is instructed to combine answers and count a total number of "yes" responses to determine whether a respondent has the symptoms required for eligibility in a depression study. At the end of the interview, the interviewer will be told on the screen whether the respondent qualifies for the study.

EXAMPLE 3.8
Calculations Programmed Into CAI

PROGRAMMER: CAI TO ENTER RESPONSES TO I-10 TO I-12.

I-10. YES TO ONE OF THE SHADED ITEMS (I1 OR I2) i.e., SAD OR LOST INTEREST?

   1   YES
   5   NO

I-11. TOTAL THE NUMBER OF "YES" RESPONSES FOR I-1 – I-9

  # YES = _____

I-11a. DOES Q11 TOTAL 5 OR MORE?

  # YES: (CAI CODE: STUDY=ELIGIBLE FOR IMPACT)
  # NO: GO TO I-13

I-12. CAI: IF I-10 = YES AND I-11 = 5+ THEN CODE I-12 (CURRENT MAJOR DEPRESSION) = YES   (1)
ELSE CODE I-12 (CURRENT MAJOR DEPRESSION) = NO   (5).

SOURCE: Project IMPACT and Center for Health Studies, Group Health Cooperative.

CAI programming can provide many useful aids for interviewing. Special instructions can be programmed to appear only if a respondent is female, for instance, or only if she reports being interested in telephone numbers of local museums exhibiting certain types of art. Formatting a questionnaire for the computer screen is a bit different from formatting print on a page. The programmer needs to consider space constraints in deciding how much can logically be displayed on one screen. The programmer also has the luxury of using not only different typefaces, type sizes, and graphics but color, which can easily be added to highlight important sections.

Question Order

Formatting questions and instructions for in-person surveys is one challenge; the order of placement of questions is another. Generally, the first items in the questionnaire should maintain respondent interest and make responding easy. The questions should usually be related to the topic of the interview as expressed in an introductory statement. This means that items concerning background or demographic factors, such as age, income, and marital status, are usually not among the first questions. When the questions flow logically from the introduction, respondents are drawn into the interview rather than being distracted and perhaps annoyed by questions they consider irrelevant (but that the surveyor may need answered at some point for statistical purposes). A smooth start also sets the tone for the rest of the interview, establishing a "rapport effect" that builds trust and enhances the respondent's willingness to participate fully in the interview. The first questions should be easy to understand and nonthreatening.

Once respondents have been drawn into the interview, complex or difficult-to-answer questions may be introduced. These should be asked before respondent fatigue becomes an issue, as responses will be less careful and likely less accurate if respondents are weary of the process. Easy-to-answer items, such as questions about demographics, are generally best placed at the end of the interview. Such questions are least likely to be affected by respondent fatigue and, because they are personal in nature, are best answered after significant rapport has been established. The order of questions intended to reconstruct a history, such as a job history, should be chronological, either forward or backward, to assist respondent recall.

When ordering questions for optimal flow, the surveyor must consider the possibility of question-order effects, or situations in which answers to certain questions may influence respondents, consciously or unconsciously, in their responding to later items. Question-order effects are a significant source of response error. Three different kinds of question-order effects, which are not always easy to anticipate or avoid, are common: consistency, fatigue, and redundancy.

CONSISTENCY EFFECT

The **consistency effect** is present when respondents feel that they must bring their responses to items into consistency with their responses to earlier items. This might occur, for example, if questions about the personal life and character of a presidential candidate precede questions about that individual's competence for office. Respondents might feel that their judgments about competence should be consistent with their earlier responses on the character questions. This context might not be present if the competence questions are asked first; the respondents might then focus on intellectual competence, for example. The consistency effect can be far more subtle than in this example, and the surveyor should always keep in mind the possibility of this effect when ordering questions. Dispersing items that respondents might be tempted to try to answer consistently, so that they are farther apart in the questionnaire, probably does not reduce the consistency effect much. Surveyors must use intuition and logic in deciding which sets of questions might influence responses to others.

FATIGUE EFFECT

The **fatigue effect** occurs when respondents begin to grow weary or bored over the course of the interview. At the beginning, respondents may give much thought to answering informatively, but later they may begin to give incomplete answers or choose not to answer difficult questions. Fatigue can set in after several related questions. Surveyors have found it useful to insert transitions and to vary question or response forms to recapture respondents' attention. Putting easy-to-answer questions at the end of the interview is also helpful.

REDUNDANCY EFFECT

The **redundancy effect** occurs when questions seem to repeat previous questions; when this happens, respondents may not answer carefully, or they may not answer at all. When items are similar but distinct in the mind of the surveyor, the questionnaire needs to be written so that the differences are clearly pointed out. For example, questions regarding smoking history may begin with something general, such as "Have you ever smoked cigarettes?" A later question, which in the mind of the surveyor is intended to distinguish current smokers from past smokers, may read, "Do you smoke cigarettes?" A respondent may not recognize the difference in the meanings of these two questions just from the context, especially if the second question does not immediately follow the first. These questions might be more clearly worded this way: "Have you ever smoked cigarettes (any time in your life)?" and "Do you currently (in the past 6 months) smoke cigarettes?"

Sometimes true redundancies cannot be avoided. For example, surveyors will sometimes use validated scales consisting of specific items to measure related characteristics. A survey might contain a scale that measures a person's level of pain and how much pain interferes with daily activities as well as another scale to measure aspects of the person's mood. Both scales might happen to contain a question about sleep problems. In one case, the context is loss of sleep due to pain, and in the other, the question concerns insomnia due to mood disorders. Still, the questions themselves can seem quite similar. Because the questions are part of validated scales (see **How to Assess and Interpret Survey Psychometrics,** Volume 8 in this series), the surveyor cannot simply delete the question from one of the scales. Instead, the surveyor should include instructions for the interviewer to acknowledge the redundancy if the respondent points it out. Interviewers should be trained to offer responses that may alleviate respondent annoyance (see Chapter 6).

Response Order

An issue similar to question order is the effect of response order on answers chosen by respondents, although response order is of greater concern with telephone interviews than with those done in person. The answers that respondents give can have more to do with the order of the options than their content. The three main sources of response-order bias are as follows:

- *Memory error:* The respondent loses track of some of the options and picks one that comes to mind easily rather than the most accurate one.

- *Primacy or recency effect:* The respondent tends to choose the first or last response regardless of content; this occurs with long lists and with rating scales (e.g., agree/disagree).

- *Response set:* The respondent tends to acquiesce or agree on items followed by rating scales (e.g., excellent/fair, approve/disapprove) regardless of his or her true feelings. This leads the respondent to tend to reply to all attitude scale questions in the same manner, regardless of the content of the questions.

The surveyor should limit the number of response categories in any given question to four or five and instruct the interviewer to read them as part of the question, to maintain continuity and a conversational tone. Lists with rating scales should be kept short (six or seven items) to reduce the likelihood of response set. When visual aids are used, longer lists can be tolerated because the interviewer can more easily probe to make sure the respondent has considered all the categories.

Question Grouping

For smooth reading and easy comprehension, questions should be grouped by topic; this allows the respondent to recognize relationships among questions. For example, questions about smoking behaviors should be grouped together, and questions about health problems should be grouped together, separately from those about smoking behavior. Although the surveyor, who has analysis purposes in mind, may see other groupings as logical (a smoking question followed by a question about a health problem thought to be related to smoking, for instance), such groupings might seem illogical and confusing to respondents and could affect response accuracy. The surveyor is better advised to group questions according to topic and then reorder them later for analysis purposes.

When moving from one group of questions to the next, the interviewer maintains the flow of the interview by reading the transition statements provided on the questionnaire. These alert the respondent that a topic change is occurring and that the next set of questions is not dependent on the previous set. A good transition statement identifies the change of context for the respondent by giving information about the next set of questions. This information can reflect a change in any of the following:

- *Response pattern:* For example, "Okay, the next set of questions has different possible answers from the one we just finished. Please answer the next set of questions with a simple yes or no."

- *Conceptual level:* For example, "The previous questions asked about what you know about gun control laws. Now I'd like to ask some questions about your feelings toward these laws."

- *Level of complexity:* For example, "Now that we have discussed these general issues, I'd like to ask you some more detailed questions on some specific topics."

A transition statement may simply tell the respondent what topic the interviewer is going to address next. The surveyor should include transition statements freely throughout the questionnaire, to give respondents a sense of movement through the interview and to establish an overall coherence among the parts of the questionnaire. Example 3.9 lists a number of samples of transition statements that might be used throughout an interview.

EXAMPLE 3.9
Sample Transition Statements

1. First, I'd like to start by asking you some general questions about yourself.

2. Now I would like to learn more about members of your family.

3. Now I am going to ask you some questions about the nonprescription medications that you may have used during the past year.

Example 3.9 continued

4. Next I would like to ask you some questions about your recent level of physical activity, and then I will ask you some questions about your activity 10 years ago.

5. Now I would like to ask you some questions about how often you are exposed to the sun and how sensitive your skin is to sun exposure.

6. Now I am going to ask you some questions about your typical eating habits in the past year.

7. Now I am going to ask you some questions about smoking.

8. Now I would like to ask you a few questions about your current and past weight. These questions are an important part of the study, so please answer as accurately as you can.

9. We are almost finished with the interview. I just have a few statistical questions that are used to group your answers with those of other people who are being interviewed.

10. This completes our interview. Thank you for taking the time to answer these questions. Do you have any comments you would like to add?

The following guidelines summarize some of the points about questionnaire construction made throughout this chapter.

Guidelines for Questionnaire Construction

Formatting Questions

- Consider the needs of the interviewer, respondent, and data entry person/programmer when formatting questions.

- Treat all questions as part of a whole, not as separate from other items.

- Arrange items and instructions for maximum readability by the interviewer. Do not break questions between pages (or CAPI screens). Provide adequate spacing in the text. Ensure that the interviewer does not have to turn pages (or scroll) back and forth during questionnaire administration.

- Use different typefaces, graphics, and spacing to distinguish questions clearly from response categories and from instructions.

- Vary response patterns and group topics as often as practical. Response set and fatigue can affect responses after six or more items of similar interest or form.

- Get input from interviewers and data entry personnel on questionnaire design.

- Precode questions whenever possible.

Ordering Questions

- Reflect the focus of the research in the first question, as stated in the introduction to the interview. Start with easy items.

- Place any complex, difficult, or sensitive questions at a point in the interview when rapport is likely to have been established and before respondent fatigue might set in.

- Place easy-to-answer questions, such as those concerning demographics, at the end of the interview to minimize inadequate responses due to respondent fatigue.
- Order questions in a way that makes sense to the respondent.
- Be aware of possible question-order effects when arranging items. For the same topic, order items from general to specific, unless respondents are expected to be unknowledgeable about the subject matter.

Grouping Questions

- Group questions according to topic. Arrange the groupings in an order that makes sense to the respondent.
- Use transition statements freely.

Pretests

The final step in preparing a questionnaire is to pretest it, to determine how well the different sections flow as a whole and whether there are unclear questions that need to be rewritten. A **pretest** is essentially a dry run in which the interviewer goes through the questionnaire with convenient respondents, some of whom should be members of the relevant population who can give realistic responses. In addition, the instrument should be pretested on interviewers and data entry personnel. These individuals can provide valuable feedback on the mechanics of the administration of the interview schedule, particularly on the quality of question flow, the accuracy and adequacy of instructions, the procedures for recording responses, the quality of the introduction, and the wording of questions. Experienced interviewers and data entry experts will have a good idea of which question orders and formats will work and which will not. Pretests also give the surveyor a chance to estimate the length of time required for administration and to experiment with sampling procedures, particularly the technique that will be used to select a member of a household. Of course, pretests also provide an excellent training opportunity for all personnel involved in the survey.

One caveat is necessary here: It is possible to pretest too much. That is, seeking advice from others can be counterproductive, particularly when those individuals want to add some questions on their favorite topics or provide very, very detailed critiques. Because designing survey questionnaires is somewhat of an art, the perfect questionnaire will never exist, and all the pretests and consulting in the world will not produce perfection. Pretests are necessary, but there comes a point when the line must be drawn and the questionnaire put into the field.

A full "dress rehearsal" of the survey with a small sample of eligible participants, called a **pilot test**, is sometimes done before a large project is put into the field. In a pilot test, interviews are done just as they will be for the full survey, with a small sample of real members of the target population in the planned interview setting. Pilot tests help surveyors determine whether all of the project procedures (not just the interview administration itself) will work as envisioned. Once the instrument is refined and finalized, the rest of the job of quality data collection is up to the interviewer.

4 How to Identify and Enlist Respondents

$\mathbf{A}$long with construction of the survey, another task that needs to be accomplished early in the start-up of a new survey is the operationalization of the chosen sampling plan. Survey staff must learn and properly implement the selected strategy. A *sample* is a portion or subset of the target population; a sample is drawn when it is impractical to survey everyone in the population. A good sample is a miniature version of the population—just like it, only smaller.

Sampling

Many surveys draw samples from some kind of a list, or sampling frame, of potential interview respondents. For example, a survey team working for a school district might randomly select respondents to interview about a new reading program from enrollment rosters at participating schools. Health researchers might use medical records from the offices of randomly selected lung specialists serving high-pollution areas to create a list of asthma patients from which to draw a sample.

Surveyors may not always find it possible or convenient to sample from lists. Instead, they may choose other methods to select candidates for participation in their surveys. For example, a large company wishing to survey employees regarding job satisfaction might randomly select offices and then randomly select desks within those offices without regard for who sits at them. The persons occupying the chosen desks would constitute the sample. As long as everyone in the company has a desk, each person has an equal chance of being chosen. A surveyor can select a sample in this way without having to compile a list of names; in this case, desks are sampled rather than people.

The criterion that every eligible person in the population of interest has an equal chance of being chosen is important in what is called *probability sampling*. There are also many methods of *nonprobability sampling*. These methods tend to be more convenient and less expensive than probability sampling methods, but surveyors who use them cannot have as much confidence that their samples fully represent the target populations. However, depending on the topic and the intended application of the survey findings, many surveys can tolerate this limitation.

Sampling is a complex topic, and a thorough examination of sampling methods is beyond the scope of this book. The principles of sound sampling are not unique to interview surveys; they are of concern to all survey researchers (for a detailed discussion of sampling issues and techniques, see **How to Sample in Surveys**, Volume 7 in this series).

There is, however, one probability sampling method that is particularly relevant to in-person surveys of the general population, and so requires brief mention here. This method is called *area probability sampling*. Area probability sampling is a very useful strategy for household sampling because it can be applied to any population that can be defined geographically. People living in a neighborhood, city, or country can be sampled this way. The target area is first divided into exhaustive, mutually exclusive subareas with identifiable boundaries, and from these a sample of subareas is randomly drawn. A list is then made of the housing units in each of these subareas, and a random sample of housing units is drawn. All of the people in the selected housing units may be included in the sample, or they may be listed and sampled separately. Recruiters and/or interviewers then approach all of the housing units in the sample in person to introduce the survey. They might conduct interviews on the spot with those who are willing to give their informed consent, or they may schedule interviews for future visits. This technique can be used for sparsely populated rural areas, for crowded downtown areas in large cities, or for any other geographic unit.

Sample Coverage

In developing the sampling plan during survey design, the surveyor must take into account considerations of internal and external validity. That is, the methods chosen for finding and screening participants should maximize the chance that people with the necessary characteristics (e.g., correct age and gender, experience with the topic of the survey) can be found and that enough eligible respondents are interviewed to provide a representative estimate of the views or experiences of the larger population. When a sample is representative of the target population, the results of the survey can be *generalized* to the entire population. Thus staff members who carry out the sampling procedures cannot alter the prescribed approach if they run into unexpected difficulties. If they cannot reach selected respondents, for example, staff members might be tempted to recruit convenient replacements. Before they can make any such changes, they need to consult the survey's designer to make sure that their "solutions" to sampling problems do not compromise the survey's generalizability.

Sample coverage is one aspect of sampling that is of particular concern because of the affects it can have on generalizability. When some members of the target population cannot be reached due to a nonrandom reason, data quality might be compromised by incomplete sample coverage. For example, individuals who are homeless or who live in cars or RVs, converted garages, or other nontraditional household settings might be overlooked by a household sampling technique. If these people are different from those who are interviewed in a way that is relevant to the survey objectives, the results will be biased; such a scenario is illustrated in Example 4.1. The incorrect conclusions drawn in such cases are said to be due to *sampling error.*

EXAMPLE 4.1
Compromised Sample Coverage

A survey is conducted to determine levels of posttraumatic stress among survivors of a serious earthquake. Two weeks after the quake, many survivors have returned to their homes, but the hardest-hit victims are still living in tents and shelters. If only traditional housing units are sampled, the individuals who are currently without homes will be skipped, and information about the stress manifestations of the hardest-hit victims, which are likely to be different from those of victims still residing in their homes, will be lost. Thus the data will be incomplete and probably biased toward lower levels of posttraumatic stress than are actually being experienced in the population of earthquake survivors.

Incomplete sample coverage can also occur when a survey has high refusal rates if refusers are different from nonrefusers in some relevant way. In a survey on teenage drinking behaviors, for example, if refusers are more likely than nonrefusers to be heavy drinkers, the results will not be representative of the entire teenage drinking population.

The process of sampling has implications for all of the initial steps of survey administration: recruitment of respondents, introduction of the study, and eligibility screening.

5 How to Administer an Interview in Person

Introductory Statement

Survey staff members follow the sampling procedure set up by the surveyor to identify possible interview respondents. Because methods vary, the means of contacting possible respondents will also vary from survey to survey. Respondents may be contacted "cold" by door-to-door recruitment, by advance telephone call, by introductory letter, or by a form of advertising. Whatever the form of contact, the survey staff member making the contact must make an introductory statement. The introductory statement, as short as it may be, has the major responsibility of establishing immediate rapport and trust between the respondent and the interviewer. The formulation of the introductory message is very important; the following checklist is intended to help guide this process.

Checklist for Preparing Introductory Statements

✓ Identify the person making the contact by his or her full name.

✓ Identify the sponsor of the survey (e.g., foundation, university, marketing firm).

✓ Explain why the request is being made, including appropriate background on the survey and what kind of information is sought.

✓ Verify that the right person, household, or telephone number has been approached.

✓ State any important conditions of the interview, such as the level of confidentiality, the voluntary nature of participation, the approximate length of the interview, and the participant's opportunity to ask questions.

✓ Describe any benefits of participation.

✓ Ask for permission to proceed with the questions (either now, if the interviewer is present, or at an agreeable future time).

It has been well documented that most interview terminations or refusals take place after the introduction but before the first question, so an interviewer will usually have an opportunity to describe the survey before the respondent decides whether or not to participate. The script for an introduction should first identify both the person making the contact and the sponsoring organization, so as to establish the survey's credibility, and then explain briefly why the request for an interview is being made. To avoid wasting both the respondent's and the recruiter's/interviewer's time, the script should next turn to verification that the correct person or location has been reached. If the right person has been found, the introduction should continue with brief details about the reason for the survey, its contents, and the conditions of the interview (e.g., confidentiality) and any benefits of participation. These details offer the respondent the opportunity to make an informed decision about participation. Finally, a courteous request for permission to proceed makes the respondent feel respected and ensures that participation is voluntary.

There is some debate among survey researchers about just how much information the introductory statement should give about the purpose of the survey. One view is that respondents should be told as little as possible about the survey objectives, because any such information might bias their response patterns. For example, if respondents know that a survey is being conducted to examine the effects of alcohol in possibly lowering the incidence of heart attacks, they might report on their alcohol consumption differently than they would if they thought the subject was alcoholism. Another view is that respondents should be well-informed, not only because they should be respected but because this can prevent them from accusing the interviewer or surveyor of malpractice or misconduct.

The amount of detail that should be provided in the introductory statement depends on the specific survey topic, its political context, potential risks to respondents if confidentiality is accidentally breached, the characteristics of the target population, and the costs to data quality from possibly biased answers. Although not always required for surveys, the process of obtaining informed consent (discussed later in this chapter) can guide the surveyor in determining how much a respondent ethically needs to know about the survey before proceeding with the interview. However, the introductory statement cannot fully cover all of this detail. It must faithfully but briefly summarize the important points, with the understanding that respondents have the right to refuse during the more formal process of obtaining informed consent.

If an incentive is being offered for participation, it should be mentioned in the introduction (e.g., "If you are eligible and choose to participate, the project will pay you $5.00 as a gesture of thanks for your time"). Incentives may be in the form of money or small gifts appropriate to the respondent group.

Example 5.1 displays two samples of introductory statements that an interviewer might deliver in person when the interview is to follow immediately.

EXAMPLE 5.1
Sample Introductory Statements

1. Hello, my name is _____, and I represent the Democratic Party. We are doing a survey to get a feel for voter opinion on gun control legislation, and I am asking people in your neighborhood for their views. I will not ask your name or record any identifying characteristics about you on the survey form, except the neighborhood where the interview took place. Your participation will make your opinions heard in Washington. The survey takes about 7 minutes to complete. Do you have any questions? May I continue?

   (SHOW IDENTIFICATION IF NECESSARY)

2. My name is _____, and I am from UCLA. We are conducting a study of the health effects of environmental pollutants, funded by the National Institutes of Health. To learn about these effects, we would like to ask you a number of questions about your health and daily activities. The

Example 5.1 continued

information that you provide will be very important in helping us understand the relationship of the environment to health and will help to guide us in making decisions in these areas in the future. Your responses will be used for statistical purposes only and will not in any way be identified with you or members of your family. If you choose to do the interview, I'd like to offer you a small gift at the end as a gesture of thanks for your time. I expect the interview to take about 15 minutes. I'd like to begin by asking you some general questions about you and all other family members living in this house. May I continue?

Comment: Note that in both of these introductory statements, the emphasis is on confidentiality information, because the physical presence of the interviewer is more threatening to privacy than a request made over the phone.

When interviewers or recruiters are recruiting in the field, it is important that they carry letters of identification certifying that they represent a legitimate organization. Interviewers and recruiters should also wear badges on which their names and the name of the sponsoring organization are clearly visible. Example 5.2 shows a sample letter of identification.

EXAMPLE 5.2
Sample Letter of Identification

(ON SURVEY CENTER LETTERHEAD)

Date
Dear Neighbor:

   This letter introduces _____, who is employed as an interviewer by Happy Families, a grassroots organization dedicated to supporting families in crisis. The interviewer is conducting a survey of your opinions regarding problems American families face and what solutions you consider appropriate. The results of the survey will be used to prepare educational materials for social workers and other professionals whose job it is to provide support to families. Your responses will be confidential. If you have questions or wish to verify the project, please feel free to call a field supervisor at 999-1234. Thank you for your help.

John Smith, Project Director

Comment: This letter contains a statement of the survey purpose, an affirmation of confidentiality, and a telephone number the respondent can call to verify that the survey is genuine. It can be helpful for such a letter to state that collect calls will be accepted or to note that the number provided is toll-free, if either is the case. If collect calls are accepted at the survey office and the line may sometimes be answered by an answering machine, the statement "Operator, we accept collect calls" should be part of the machine's outgoing message.

Advance Letters and Precalls

Of course, potential participants do not always receive in-person introductions to surveys. Instead, they might receive **advance letters** (or **preletters**), when a sampling list with addresses is available, or **precalls** (introductory calls made to describe and schedule interviews, not to administer them). By reducing the element of surprise and increasing the time that potential respondents have to think about participating, advance letters and precalls can reduce refusal rates and increase data quality. These tools can also demonstrate the authenticity of the project, so that a potential respondent does not assume that a sales pitch is coming.

Using the following guidelines can help to ensure that an introductory letter makes an appropriate impression on the respondent.

Guidelines for Preparing Advance Letters

- Print the letter on the survey organization's letterhead.

- If the sample size is manageable, use a personal salutation (e.g., Dear Mr. Jones) and sign each letter individually in ink.

- Date the letter to coincide with the mailing. An undated letter will appear to be less personal.

- Include an introductory statement regarding a future call or visit to conduct an interview. Mention timing of the contact, how the respondent was sampled and chosen, and whether someone else in the household might ultimately be interviewed.

- Describe the survey topic without being intimidating.

- Guarantee whatever level of confidentiality is possible.

- Give an honest estimate of the time required to complete the interview.

- Convey the importance of respondent views for valid results and potential impact.

It is important that an advance letter convey the survey's legitimacy through appropriate identification of the sponsor and the source of the survey. Printing the letter on the survey center's or the sponsor's letterhead helps provide this identification. It is also helpful if the advance letter presents as personal an appeal to the potential respondent as possible. Each person who receives a preletter should feel that he or she has been singled out for this interview and that his or her opinion is crucial to the study. Personalization of preletters through individualized salutations, original (not "rubber-stamp") signatures, and individually typed or printed envelopes has been shown to stimulate response, particularly from somewhat reluctant respondents. Of course, personalization is expensive to implement and cannot always be done for very large samples.

Including information about the timing of a future contact in the preletter helps the potential respondent to anticipate the visit and provides him or her with an opportunity to consider whether to participate in the survey. As with introductory statements in general, other details included in the preletter—about sampling, survey topic, confidentiality, and so forth—give the recipient the information he or she needs to make a decision about participating. An advance letter may be written as though it comes directly from the survey group (see Example 5.3), or it may take the form of an endorsement from a supporter of or collaborator in the survey whom the potential respondent is likely to trust (see Example 5.4).

EXAMPLE 5.3
Advance Letter: In-Home Interview

(ON SURVEY CENTER LETTERHEAD)

Date
Mr. Thomas Edison
222 Your Street
Your Town, USA

Dear Mr. Edison:

In the next few weeks, you will be called by an interviewer representing your local school board about an extremely important survey on the use of standardized testing among elementary school children. Your opinions are vital to determining whether and how such testing should be implemented and paid for. Your participation and cooperation are important so that the results of the research can be statistically valid. You are one of 950 individuals chosen by scientific methods to participate in this survey. We got your telephone number and address from the Hill-Donnelly Criss-Cross Directory, which matches listed telephone numbers and addresses. Your responses will be completely confidential.

We are not attempting to sell you anything; we only want your opinions. If you wish to verify the authenticity of the survey, or if you have any questions about the purpose of this project, you can call me directly at 888-4321.

When our interviewer calls you within the next few days, we would appreciate your making an appointment for an interview. We would like to conduct this interview in your home, and it will last approximately 45 minutes. Thank you for your consideration.

Sincerely,
Lisa Jones, Ph.D.
Project Director
Survey Center

Example 5.3 continued

Comment: This advance letter, which is printed on the survey center's letterhead, is intended to inform a potential respondent that a request for an in-person interview is going to be made by telephone.

EXAMPLE 5.4
Advance Letter From a Trusted Collaborator

(ON PHYSICIAN'S LETTERHEAD)

Dear Ms. Smith:

I have been asked by the University of California to help them in a national study about the overall health of Americans. Many individuals from all parts of the country are being invited to help in this study.

In order to get correct information about the health of Americans, I need your cooperation. Because this study is important, I am asking my patients to take part in it. You can help by answering a number of questions about your health. A project staff member will come to your home, or some other place if you prefer, to ask you some questions. The interview should take about an hour of your time.

The information you give will be kept strictly confidential. When your interview is finished, your name will be removed from the questionnaire. The answers you give will be combined with the answers given by all other persons interviewed and used for scientific study.

Please drop the enclosed postcard in the mail so that a member of the study staff may call you and answer any questions you may have and also arrange the best time and place for your interview. Or, if you prefer, the project staff or I would be glad to answer any questions. The

Example 5.4 continued

staff can be reached at (310) 555-1234 (CALL COLLECT IF THIS IS OUT OF YOUR AREA).

I urge you to participate in this important study by the University of California conducted under the sponsorship of the National Institutes of Health.

Sincerely,

James Jones, M.D.

Comment: When confidentiality is of great concern, as in the case of having chosen a respondent from a medical records review in which sensitive information may be involved, the advance letter might come from a physician the respondent knows and trusts. If the physician is part of the survey team or clearly endorses the project, the letter serves to legitimate the study and make the respondent more comfortable about revealing personal information.

Similar to advance letters, precalls serve to inform potential respondents of their selection for interview and should include the same basic information about the survey. A future visit for an interview can be scheduled during the precall if the person consents. When the actual interview is conducted, the interviewer's script for the opening comments might refer back to the precall. The script for a precall should cover the same basic content as an in-person introduction or advance letter.

Advance letters, precalls, and introductory statements made in person all serve to entice potential respondents to participate in a survey. An interviewer must be certain, however, before proceeding with an interview, that the person contacted is *eligible* to be a respondent.

Eligibility Screen

In the course of introducing the survey, the recruiter/interviewer must determine whether the potential respondent is actually eligible to participate. This is accomplished using an **eligibility screen**—that is, a set of questions designed to screen out individuals who do not meet the survey's eligibility criteria. In surveys of the general public, researchers are often interested in polling the views of individuals with specific characteristics, such as people who are registered voters or people who most often do the grocery shopping for their families. If the survey respondents are grouped on a sampling list that was generated according to inclusion criteria (e.g., mothers of children with speech impairments who have received speech therapy at a local clinic), the interviewer presumably knows the name of the desired respondent and can ask for that person directly. This does not necessarily ensure eligibility, however; there may be other criteria that need to be reviewed with the respondent directly (e.g., the surveyor may be interested only in mothers who also have at least one other child in the household). Interviewers must be trained in the importance of eligibility criteria and cautioned not to accept convenient substitutes (as substitution can affect sample coverage).

The eligibility screen consists of one or more questions designed to determine whether the potential respondent has the characteristics the surveyor considers important. The interviewer should ask these questions after establishing rapport during the introductory phase and before beginning the interview. This timing is ideal because potential respondents are more likely to give truthful answers to eligibility questions if they already trust that the interviewer's purpose is legitimate, and resources are not wasted interviewing ineligible respondents whose data will have to be disregarded.

Example 5.5 presents a sample of an eligibility screen that is part of a survey's introductory script. The surveyor in this case is screening potential participants at a beach and wants to limit findings to a single day of contact with the water during a specified period of time. Thus anyone who may come back to the beach during that period is not eligible.

EXAMPLE 5.5
Sample Eligibility Screen

Hi. I'm with the Southern California Beaches Health Survey. We are here at the beach today asking families about their contact with the water. In about 10 days, another person from the survey or I will phone those who talk to us today. We will ask some follow-up questions about the water. We will also ask some health questions at that time. Are you willing to answer some questions today? Are you here with your family? (IF YES, PROCEED WITH ELIGIBILITY QUESTIONS.)

Have you or anyone in your household been swimming or playing in the water at this beach today?

Yes → CONTINUE TO Q2
No   → THANK AND END INTERVIEW

Not including (3-day survey period), do you think you or anyone in your household will return to this beach in the next 10 days?

Yes, we will all return
→ THANK AND END INTERVIEW

Yes, some of us will return
→ CONTINUE **ONLY** FOR THOSE WHO WILL **NOT** RETURN BUT WHO **HAVE BEEN IN THE WATER**

No, none of us will return
→ CONTINUE INTERVIEW FOR ENTIRE HOUSEHOLD

SOURCE: Adapted from the Santa Monica Beach Study Pilot.

Sometimes a single contact attempt will reach more than one eligible respondent, especially in population surveys for which there is no "list." It can be necessary to sample within a household or living unit, particularly if an individual, not a household, is the unit of analysis. Because households can be clusters of eligible respondents, it is necessary to sample within the cluster if a random probability sample is desired. In some cases, it is necessary to get responses only from any members of the household who are familiar with the survey topic. It is also not necessary to implement a within-household selection procedure if the eligibility screen is directed at a very specific member—say, a female over the age of 55 or a member of the household who plays golf, cares for an elder, or has a disability. If such criteria are defined, they can be incorporated into the eligibility script. If they are not defined, interviewers can be instructed to use one of several selection procedures to choose from among several eligible household members. These are discussed only briefly here (for more exhaustive reviews, see the sources listed in the "Suggested Readings" section at the end of this book).

Interviewers may be instructed to select the *first eligible* respondent to come to the telephone or answer the door when resources are limited and time may be a factor. In such a case, the interviewer verifies that the potential respondent meets minimum qualification criteria (e.g., "over the age of 18" or "lived in household for more than 3 months") and then conducts the interview. This selection process produces a "convenience" sample that is not a probability design. Generalization of the findings from such a sample to the larger population can be made only with some caution. This technique oversamples females, particularly when contact is made by telephone, as women tend to be the ones who answer the phone in many households. Some survey researchers implement a male-female alternate selection process, but this assumes that the distribution of gender is known and that substitution does not compromise the distribution of population characteristics.

Another type of selection procedure calls for the enumeration of household members. In this technique, the interviewer asks for a listing of all members of a household by age, gender, and relation to head of household, and then chooses a respondent from among them. This technique is time-consuming and more demanding of interviewers than other techniques. It also produces higher-than-normal refusal rates, because many people resist describing the composition of their households to strangers.

In another technique, the interviewer asks for the person in the household who had the most recent birthday or will have the next birthday. The request for birthday information is not threatening to the respondent, and the probability of selection is preserved because it is assumed that the distribution of birthdays in a population is random, not systematic or patterned in any way. The interviewer reads from a script such as the following:

"We need to be sure we give every adult a chance to be interviewed for this study. Thinking only of adults in your household, that is, persons over the age of 18, which one had the most recent birthday? (or will have the next birthday)? Would you be that person?"

IF YES, CONTINUE INTERVIEW
IF NO, "May I speak to that person?"
(REPEAT INTRODUCTION)

Very often, the person answering the telephone or initially responding to an in-person interview request is also the eligible respondent—that is, has the next or most recent birthday. In practice, the use of "most recent birthday" is preferable to "next birthday" because it is easier for people to recall who recently had a birthday than to figure out who will have one in the near future.

Questions From Respondents

At some time while the interviewer is presenting the introductory statement and the eligibility screen, the potential respondent or others in the household are very likely to ask questions regarding the survey to determine whether it is legitimate and to help them decide whether or not to participate. Although some respondent questions might come up at the end of the interview or even during its administration, most will be asked near the beginning of the contact. All interviewers in a given survey study must answer such questions in a consistent manner, and they must be trained not to add information that could bias respondents' answers. The surveyor should develop **recommended responses** (sometimes called *fallback statements*) for interviewers to give for all of the questions that respondents and potential respondents are most likely to ask.

Interviewers need to be very familiar with these standardized responses and should keep lists of them readily available as memory backups during interviews. They should be instructed to call on a supervisor to respond to any respondent questions they cannot answer. When no supervisor is present, which is the case during most in-person interviews, the interviewer should get the respondent's telephone number and tell the respondent that a supervisor will call soon with an answer to the question.

Following are some of the kinds of questions most frequently asked by respondents:

- How did you get my name [telephone number, address]?
- Whom do you represent?
- Who is sponsoring this survey?
- Will you use my name?
- How will you use my answers?

- Will this cost me anything, or will I be paid for my participation?

- What will happen if I don't participate?

Depending on the topic of the specific survey being conducted, the surveyor can usually anticipate other likely respondent questions (e.g., in a survey of satisfaction with health care, respondents might want to know whether their doctors will have access to their responses or names). Example 5.6 lists some possible questions that respondents might have regarding a nuclear power survey and the prepared answers supplied to interviewers.

EXAMPLE 5.6
Standardized Responses to Respondent Questions About a Nuclear Power Survey

What is the Center for Survey Research?

This is a research unit of the University of Nevada, Las Vegas, designed for the purpose of conducting public opinion polls and surveys on various social, political, and economic issues.

Who is paying for this research?

This is a cooperative project funded by the Sagebrush Alliance and the Department of Sociology at UNLV.

Who or what is the Sagebrush Alliance?

The Sagebrush Alliance is a community group concerned with the evaluation of the impact of environmental changes on the quality of life of residents of the state of Nevada.

Example 5.6 continued

How did you get my name?

We do not have or need your name. We are just visiting people in your neighborhood at random.

How do I know this is confidential?

We do not have your name. We are interested only in combining the responses of the 400 or so persons who will be interviewed. Individual responses will not be singled out. All of us working on this project are required to follow certain procedures and guidelines developed to protect the identity of persons who respond to the survey.

How will the results be used?

The information generated by this survey will be used by students in research methods classes. The results will also be made available to policy makers in the community to help them know and understand what county residents think about the nature and use of nuclear energy and about other issues.

What is the purpose of the survey?

This is a general survey of the public on a number of community issues including nuclear power. The study is designed to learn more about the public's opinions and perceptions.

How long will this take?

The interview will take about 10 minutes. You can end the interview at any time, but we hope you will not.

Teaching interviewers how to deal with questions about the conditions and intent of the survey is an important part of interviewer training, especially for field interviewers who cannot be monitored closely.

Dealing With Refusals

In any survey, despite a convincing introduction and eligibility procedure, some respondents will refuse to participate. They may be suspicious of strangers or of how their responses will be used. They may even feel hostile toward the organization conducting the survey (such as "the government") or toward the topic of the survey. They may fear that they are being set up for a sales pitch or "con game." Some may just have no interest in participating, may not feel well enough, or truly be too busy.

The use of advance calls and preletters sometimes helps to lower refusal rates. A knowledgeable, courteous verbal approach can also help, especially if the recruiter/interviewer is well versed in respectful responses to common objections (see Chapter 6). It is important that recruiters not push so hard that potential respondents adamantly refuse at the first contact. After a refusal, recontact on a different day, possibly by a different staff member, may catch an individual at a more approachable moment. The first contact with any potential respondent should be well documented, so that the next contact can take into account what happened before. Sometimes a reluctant respondent will come through when approached a second time. Of course, sometimes a recruiter must take no for an answer. This too must be documented, so that the individual is not contacted again.

Informed Consent

When respondents participate in surveys that deal with sensitive subjects, they may be at risk of some discomfort or harm if confidentiality should be broken somehow. Such surveys, as well as those conducted in conjunction with some other forms of data collection, such as medical record review or provision of specimens (e.g., blood samples), require formal approval by institutional review boards (IRBs). IRBs are committees of individuals who review the protocols, questionnaires, and confidentiality provisions of planned surveys as well as any other pertinent information to determine whether the plans are ethical and the surveys may proceed. Most organizations that do surveys frequently have their own IRBs. Small groups conducting one-time surveys may need to create IRBs or submit their survey proposals to the IRBs of larger available organizations in their communities, such as universities.

After reviewing a proposal, an IRB may determine (a) that the survey is exempt from the need for approval because the risks are minimal or there are no risks; (b) that the risks are minimal, but the survey team should draft an informative letter to be given to participants to read and keep; (c) that full review and formal **informed consent** procedures are required; or (d) that the survey may not be implemented because the risks are too great. In the case of the last kind of finding, the survey team may rethink the study procedures and submit the new plans for IRB approval as appropriate. When the IRB makes the second and third kinds of determinations, this means that survey respondents are entitled to know the following:

- What procedures will be followed and their purpose
- What, if any, discomforts or risks participation might involve
- Whom to contact for inquiries about the project
- That participation is voluntary and may be withdrawn at any time without penalty
- How confidentiality will be maintained
- What the benefits of participation might be

When a survey requires the informed consent of participants, the survey team must develop an informed consent form according to specific criteria and get the form approved by the IRB. The information that an informed consent form must cover generally includes the elements listed above, but individual IRBs often have their own particular requirements and preferred formats. It is generally advised that the language of the informed consent form be kept simple, about sixth- to eighth-grade level, depending on the target population. Example 5.7 illustrates what an informed consent form for a sensitive survey topic might look like.

EXAMPLE 5.7
Sample Informed Consent Form

Informed Consent
A STUDY OF ALCOHOL USE IN OLDER PERSONS

Dear Potential Participant,

You are being asked to participate in a research project conducted by Options for Older Adults, a private support organization providing service to individuals over the age of 60. This information sheet will give you details of the project to see if you might want to join. We are asking individuals who are over 60 to be part of the project. You can quit the project at any time, and you are not required to answer any questions that you feel uncomfortable about answering. Your participation is completely voluntary. You may withdraw your consent at any time.

What is the project about?

Older persons may become more sensitive to alcohol, and alcohol also interacts with medications used by older persons. The purpose of this project is to find out what role alcohol consumption plays in the lives of older people and how we can educate people to drink safely.

Example 5.7 continued

What are you being asked to do?

If you want to participate in the project, we will ask you to participate in an interview. The interview can be done in your home or at the study office [location], according to your preference. The interview will take about 30 minutes to complete. It will ask questions about how much you drink and why.

Are there any risks or discomforts?

The only risks of participating in this project are the inconvenience of taking the time to answer the questions and the possibility that some of the questions may worry or embarrass you. There are no medical procedures involved.

What are the possible benefits?

The benefits of the study to you directly, if any, are not known yet, but the investigators hope that the survey will help benefit people in the future.

Will my privacy be protected?

All the information that you report in the interview is confidential and will be used only for the purposes of the survey project. Your name will not be recorded or used.

Whom do I contact if I have further questions?

You may call [Jane Smith], the project director, at (XXX) XXX-XXXX.

If you have any further questions, comments, or concerns about the study or the informed consent process, you may write or call [the organization's] Office for Protection of Research Subjects, Box 234, Los Angeles, CA 99999, (XXX) XXX-XXXX.

Example 5.7 continued

A copy of this informed consent statement will be given to you to keep.
If you wish to join the project, please sign below.

Name _____

Date _____

SOURCE: Adapted from the Alcohol-Related Problems Survey Project, Arlene
Fink Associates.

Once consent has been obtained, the interview can be administered. Consent forms can be mailed to respondents in advance with preletters, or consent can be obtained over the phone or in person right before the interview is begun. Often it is advisable for interviewers to summarize the key points in the consent form verbally, or to read the form to respondents to make sure they fully understand everything. After a respondent has signed the consent form, the interviewer retains the original (to return to the survey center with the completed questionnaire) and gives the respondent a copy to keep for future reference.

Enrollment

More often than not, individuals will agree to be interviewed. In many cases, a person becomes a participant simply by proceeding with the interview. All that may be necessary to "enroll" the respondent in the survey project are the creation of a log entry and the assignment of an ID number. For projects that have more complicated protocols, however, enrollment may involve further details, especially if the respondent will need to be recontacted at intervals for additional interviews (as in longitudinal studies). Example 5.8 displays a sample of the kind of enrollment form that may need to be completed for each respondent in such studies. Once respondent permission has been obtained and any other formalities have been taken care of, interviewing can begin.

EXAMPLE 5.8
Sample Enrollment Form for Tracking Respondents for Future Interviews

Enrollment Form

Enrollment ID #: ___ ___ ___ - ___ ___ ___ ___ ___
Interview Date: ___/___/___
Study ID #: ___ ___ - ___ ___ ___

Contact Information:
Name (last, first): _____
Address: _____
_____
_____

Phone: _____

Best times to call (e.g., mornings, afternoons, evenings, weekends): _____
_____

SSN: _____ (for incentive payments)

Birth date: __ __ / __ __ / __ __ __ __

Gender: __ Male __ Female

Two Friends or Relatives Study May Contact
  in Case of Move:
Name: _____
Relationship: _____
Phone: _____
Address: _____

Example 5.8 continued

Name: _____
Relationship: _____
Phone: _____
Address: _____

Notes:

1. Fax both sides of enrollment form to Survey Coordinating Center.

2. Back up all interview data.

3. Transmit data to Coordinating Center per instructions in recruiter manual.

SOURCE: Adapted from Project IMPACT.

Comment: This form is designed for the collection of information that will help the survey team to locate the respondent for future interviews. The names, phone numbers, and addresses of two contacts are taken down (with the respondent's permission) in case the respondent is no longer reachable at the current phone number when the next interview is due. The respondent's social security number is recorded if checks will need to be made out to compensate the respondent after each interview. Birth date and gender are recorded as identifiers.

Interview Administration

The administration of the interview involves five basic elements:

1. *Starting the interview:* The interviewer needs to engage the respondent with a personable but professional manner from the start. Depending on the location of the interview, the interviewer and respondent sit

down in an appropriate space and the interviewer begins the questioning. If the interview is being conducted in the respondent's home, the interviewer should suggest that they choose a place for the interview that affords privacy and is away from the activities of other family members, such as at the kitchen table. The interviewer and respondent should generally sit facing each other at a distance of about 3 feet, although this may be modified according to the respondent's cultural context.

2. *Using the questionnaire:* The interviewer must take a tone of conversational neutrality in working through the questionnaire, reading questions exactly as written and keeping personal opinions and interpretations out of the interview. The interviewer needs to use **probes** (methods for eliciting additional information when a given response is unclear) and **prompts** (statements intended to clarify the meaning of a question when the respondent has not understood it) properly. Special probes and prompts are scripted into the body of the questionnaire for the interviewer to read as appropriate. General probes that the interviewer can use with any question, such as simply repeating a question or asking for more detail, are not scripted; rather, the interviewer learns to use these in training (see Chapter 6). If the interview is done in CAPI, the interviewer must learn how to use the computer and the CAPI program well, so that he or she doesn't get tied up with figuring out how to enter answers and move to the next question. Whether the interview is done on paper or by computer, the interviewer needs to be familiar with how to code responses correctly and how to skip to the appropriate next question without breaking flow. When a respondent gives a narrative response to an open-ended question or makes a statement to clarify a confusing response, the interviewer should record the com-

ments verbatim. (On a paper questionnaire, the interviewer can write these comments in the margins. In CAPI, the interviewer can pull up a text box to type the comments in by pressing a special key; hitting another key returns the interviewer to the body of the interview.)

3. *Working with the respondent:* An important aspect of interview administration is the interviewer's proper guidance of the respondent. Most people are not used to the structure of a standardized interview and may require guidance in answering questions "usefully." Although the interviewer is not free to help the respondent formulate responses, he or she can provide certain cues that will help the respondent recognize when an answer matches the intent of the question. The interviewer may use a neutral reinforcing statement, such as "That's helpful to know," when an answer is complete and clear.

4. *Ending the interview:* When the interview is complete, it is generally best for the interviewer to thank the respondent and depart expeditiously. Although a small amount of conversation is appropriate at this point, professionalism can be compromised if the interviewer becomes too chatty. If an incentive (payment or gift) is to be given to the respondent, it is usually best to do this after the questioning has been completed. If an additional interview needs to be planned, the interviewer and respondent can set a time and date for a next visit before the interviewer leaves.

5. *Quality control:* An important aspect of interviewing is documentation. All of the interviewer's coding marks and notes need to be decipherable by those who must work with the data later. As soon as possible after leaving the respondent, the interviewer needs to go back through the questionnaire to look for and correct any

errors or illegible notes; this is called **editing** the interview. Later, a reviewer or supervisor will do another check to make sure all of the documentation seems correct and logical.

Chapter 6 provides greater detail about interview administration and how survey researchers should train interviewers to perform their tasks well.

6

How to Select, Train, and Supervise Interviewers

Successful survey data collection is the result of a well-designed questionnaire artfully administered by skillful interviewers. As mentioned in previous chapters, data quality can be compromised when interviewers use biased questioning styles or improper clarification techniques, or when they record responses inaccurately, ask questions out of sequence or skip questions, or fail to establish proper rapport with respondents. Good interviewers always use unbiased questioning techniques, proper clarifications, and correct question order, and they are careful to establish rapport with respondents. Good interviewing is the result of quality training combined with compatible natural abilities on the part of the trainee.

Roles

A skilled interviewer enhances the collection of reliable and valid data through artful application of standardized interviewing procedures. Successful interviewers use these procedures to perform three major tasks:

- *Maximization of the number of completed interviews:* Successful interviewers keep refusals and early terminations of interviews to a minimum.

- *Motivation of thoughtful participation by respondents:* Successful interviewers motivate respondents by delivering the introductory statement as written, answering respondent questions, and engaging respondents in the interview process.

- *Administration of the questionnaire:* Successful interviewers ask all questions in the correct order, record all answers clearly, and probe incomplete responses.

To perform these major tasks well, interviewers must possess a combination of specific abilities, knowledge, and skills.

ABILITIES

Interviewers must have certain abilities, or underlying capacities, to perform the basic tasks of the job without special training. An interviewer must, for example, be able to read and comprehend the interview, record the responses, work during hours when respondents can be reached, and, in the case of in-person interviewing, get to the interview site. Interviewers need to have the following basic abilities:

- The ability to speak clearly and use correct grammar in the language of the interview

- The ability to read in the language of the interview to deliver written statements and question sequences without pauses and to understand written instructions

- The ability to write in the language of the interview to record verbatim responses accurately with proper spelling

- The ability to recall responses long enough to record them accurately

- The ability to perform several tasks simultaneously: read questions, record answers, and follow instructions

- The ability to work flexible hours, usually including evenings and weekends

- The ability to travel to the interview site

- The ability to participate in one or more formal training sessions to acquire specific knowledge and skills required for performing interviews

- The ability to judge nonverbal and verbal cues that respondents give, to sense when reinforcement and clarification are needed

- The ability to exercise self-discipline and regulate their own verbal and nonverbal behaviors so as not to influence responses improperly

KNOWLEDGE

Interviewers need to master particular principles and information in order to administer interviews well. Trainers experienced in survey administration can teach interviewers the knowledge they will need for specific surveys during formal training sessions. In general, interviewers need to have an understanding of the following:

- The role of the interviewer in conducting surveys

- The importance of maintaining neutrality during interviews

- Information about the survey project sufficient to answer respondent questions

- The objectives of the survey
- Techniques for minimizing refusal rates
- The principle of confidentiality and its importance for protecting the identities of respondents and the integrity of data collection
- Procedures for contacting respondents and introducing the survey
- Correct procedures for asking questions
- Techniques of probing during an interview
- Procedures for recording answers
- Rules for handling interpersonal aspects of the interview
- Administrative procedures related to project operation, such as filling out contact sheets, mileage logs, reimbursement forms, and time sheets

SKILLS

Skills, or the capabilities to do specific tasks well, may arise from talent, practice, training, or (usually) a combination thereof. A skilled interviewer performs the tasks of the job well. Interviewers need the following skills:

- The skill to initiate and maintain a conversation with a stranger
- The skill to respond professionally to unexpected questions and situations
- The skill to remain neutral by keeping personal opinions out of the interview process
- The skill to motivate reluctant respondents to participate in the interview while demonstrating respect
- The skill to deliver the questionnaire in a flowing, conversational manner

- The skill to probe incomplete responses in an unbiased manner for more useful results

- The skill to move correctly through the skip patterns in the questionnaire

- The skill to record responses and notes correctly

- The skill to keep accurate logs

- The skill to edit interviews for errors

- The skill to maintain confidentiality

Selection Process

Interviewing is a difficult job. Selecting interviewers for a particular survey involves recruiting applicants, evaluating their qualifications for becoming good interviewers (reviewing résumés and conducting job interviews), and offering positions to the most qualified candidates. For a small survey with few resources, interviewers may be chosen from among existing staff at the organization conducting the survey; a larger operation with a bigger budget may use internal staff or may formally recruit candidates from outside. In either case, it is important that individuals with the most promising characteristics and abilities be chosen for the task of interviewing, because, as stated previously, not everyone has the potential to be a good interviewer.

JOB DESCRIPTION

The first step in identifying potential interviewers is the development of a job description that lists the tasks and duties an interviewer must perform on a specific survey project as well as the abilities, knowledge, and skills required to execute those tasks and duties. The level of detail necessary to provide in the job description varies from project to project. In general, a good job description contains four key sections:

- *Summary statement:* A brief description of the purpose of the survey and the role of the interviewer

- *Supervision:* A description of how performance will be monitored and evaluated and what level of independence is expected

- *Duties and tasks:* A list of the components of the work the interviewer will be assigned (e.g., screening respondents, by telephone or in person; administering questionnaires; filling out forms)

- *Abilities, knowledge, and skills:* A list of the qualifications—that is, what a good interviewer must know and be able to do—in specific terms, stating which are required at the outset and which the interviewer will be trained to do after hire

A good job description tells prospective interviewers what to expect of the job and what will be expected of them if they are hired. A job description such as the one in Example 6.1 can be used to advertise the availability of interviewer positions and recruit applicants. When screening applicants, the survey researcher should match the abilities, knowledge, and skills shown on applicants' résumés with the abilities, knowledge, and skills required for the particular interviewer position. The qualifications listed in the job description can also be used to formulate job interview questions about applicants' suitability for the position. Even if interviewers are being chosen from existing staff at an organization implementing its own survey, candidates should be screened and interviewed.

EXAMPLE 6.1
Sample Job Description

Summary Statement   The Acme Grocery Company requires interviewers to administer an in-person survey of customer satisfaction. The survey will be administered to customers of selected Acme grocery stores in the greater Los Angeles area during their regular shopping time. Shoppers will receive a $5 grocery gift certificate for participation in the 15-minute interview. Acme will use the survey results to improve product selection and enhance marketing strategies.

Supervision   Under general supervision of an outside survey team, interviewers will approach and survey shoppers in grocery store locations. The survey team will train interviewers in all procedures, monitor and evaluate completed interviews for accuracy and completeness, and provide feedback as necessary.

Duties and Tasks   Interviewers will approach shoppers according to a specific selection procedure. Interviewers will enlist shopper cooperation using memorized scripts and obtain questionnaire responses from those who agree to participate. Questionnaires will be administered by computer-assisted personal interview (CAPI) using laptop computers at a small station set up near the entrance of the store. Interviewers will record responses and edit completed interviews for errors before submission to the survey team. Interviewers will track and distribute $5 grocery gift certificates to shoppers who complete the survey.

Example 6.1 continued

Abilities, Knowledge, and Skills   Interviewers must have good reading, writing, and speaking abilities to read questionnaire items and record responses in English. They must also be available to conduct interviews during evening and weekend hours and to attend a half-day training session. General computer literacy is required. Skills for selecting participants, enlisting customer cooperation, maintaining confidentiality, and administering questionnaires using CAPI technology will be taught.

The best interviewers are those who have a certain intuition or talent for dealing with people in an engaging and professional manner. Intuition and talent are not measurable qualities. They surface as trained interviewers begin testing their skills in practice sessions and on the job.

Training

Once interviewers have been selected and have accepted job offers, they must be trained. The depth and detail of interviewer training materials will vary with the survey project. Training procedures usually include some combination of the following elements: a training manual; lectures, presentations, and discussions; practice; observation; and field training.

Training manual. The training manual is an important document, both for teaching interviewers how to do their jobs and for interviewers to use as a reference on the job. The manual provides context for the interviewer, describes the interviewer's obligations, and outlines interviewing techniques. The next major section of this chapter is devoted to a detailed discussion of the contents of the training manual.

Lectures, presentations, and discussions. Whenever possible, training procedures should include formal training sessions. During such sessions, the material in the training manual is presented orally by a trainer who is experienced in survey work and interviewing. Important skills and a model interview are demonstrated. A later section of this chapter focuses on the purposes and content of interviewer training sessions.

Practice. The training sessions should provide trainees with ample opportunities for supervised practice. After seeing an interview demonstrated, trainees should take turns role-playing the parts of both the interviewer and the respondent. Trainees should also interview the trainer, who can improvise difficult or unusual responses. The trainer should observe the role-playing and give direct feedback to trainees. If available, volunteer respondents (e.g., other survey staff members) could be brought in for trainees to interview after practicing among themselves. Trainees should be encouraged to perform as many simulated interviews (with friends, relatives, neighbors) as they can to become familiar with the survey instrument. Each trainee can also conduct a mock in-person interview of the trainer for further training and ultimately for testing purposes.

Observation. If a new group of interviewers is being trained for an ongoing project, it can be useful for the trainer to have them observe veteran interviewers on the job. This is possible if respondents are willing to give permission to have their interviews observed, but the survey team must weigh the advantage this method has for training interviewers against the possibility that the trainees' presence will influence respondents' answers. An alternative approach would be to have trainees listen to audiotapes of interviews or watch interviews on videotape. (If the survey plan includes recording a few real interviews for training purposes, this may require IRB approval and the development of a separate consent form for participants that specifically describes how the tapes will be used and how long they will be kept.)

Field training. The final phase of interviewer training involves on-the-spot feedback in the field. A supervisor or trainer accompanies the novice interviewer to the interview site in the field (i.e., to the respondent's home or wherever the interview is to be conducted) and observes the interview (with the respondent's permission). The supervisor or trainer stays quietly in the background and takes notes on how well the interviewer delivers the questions, how well he or she probes and prompts the respondent, whether the interviewer remains neutral, and so on. The supervisor or trainer then provides feedback to the interviewer—not in front of the respondent, but as soon after the interview as feasible (for example, in the car on the way to the next scheduled interview). Field training can be extremely useful because it confronts interviewers with real situations they may not have imagined would arise, and trainers can give them immediate input.

After completion of training, interviewers should not be allowed to interview real respondents on their own until they have been tested and "certified" by a trainer or an experienced interviewer. For this test, the actual survey instrument should be used in a realistic simulation. For example, if the interview will be administered using CAPI, the interviewer should be tested using the CAPI version of the instrument on the type of computer to be used in the field, not a paper printout. The trainer uses a predetermined script and plays the respondent in the mock interview. During the interview, the trainer observes and evaluates the trainee's reading of the questions as well as use of appropriate probing, prompting, and skipping, but does not give feedback until after the entire interview is complete. The trainer also reviews the trainee's recording of responses, checking to see whether confusing responses that were probed led to accurate response choices and whether text notes were recorded verbatim. If the trainer is satisfied that the trainee has acquired the necessary skills, the trainee can move on to interviewing actual respondents. If the trainer is not satisfied, he or she provides specific feedback to the trainee and offers more practice until the trainee gets the hang of the process.

The Training Manual

Although many of the instructions given to interviewers are very similar from survey to survey, details and context vary. Most surveys require the development of project-specific training manuals. The sample table of contents in Example 6.2 shows the general topics that are usually covered in an interviewer training manual. Most of these elements are discussed briefly below.

EXAMPLE 6.2
Sample Table of Contents
of an Interviewer Training Manual

Description of the Survey
Introduction to Survey Methods
Interviewing Techniques and Guidelines
    Preparing for the Interview
    Beginning the Interaction/Dealing With Refusals
    Establishing the Environment
    Asking the Questions
    Probing
    Clarifying
    Reinforcing the Respondent
    Closing the Interaction

The Interviewer's Responsibilities
    Contacting Respondents
    Confidentiality

Example 6.2 continued

How to Use the Interview/How to Use CAPI
Special Procedures
Use of Technology
Editing the Interview

Appendices
Introductory Script
Question-by-Question Specifications
    for Interview Questions
Sample Interview
Forms and Administrative Procedures
Interview Summary Form
Control Sheet
Call Record
Time Sheets
Sample Name Badge

SOURCE: Adapted from Kaiser/UCLA Sigmoid Study.

DESCRIPTION OF THE SURVEY

This section of the manual introduces the interviewer to the purpose of the survey in some detail, imparting information on the greater context within which interviews will be conducted. It may provide helpful background details such as descriptions of the target population, the sampling procedures used, and the objectives of the survey, and may give the names of key individuals involved in the project, such as survey coordinators and collaborators.

INTRODUCTION TO SURVEY METHODS

This section outlines the basic steps of conducting surveys, with emphasis on the interviewer's place in the process. The steps described include data collection, coding, and data entry (if the interviews are not to be administered by computer), and may also include brief statements about data cleaning, analysis, and reporting of results. The key role that interviewers play in data collection should be highlighted. This section may also describe the flow of data through the survey office, from interviewing through computerized data management, and the nature of the supervision to be provided for the project as a whole.

INTERVIEWING TECHNIQUES AND GUIDELINES

This section gives the interviewer important information about how to conduct interviews by breaking the process down into steps such as those described below.

Preparing for the Interview

The manual should give specific information about how the interviewer should prepare to conduct interviews. For example, the interviewer should review and practice all survey materials and procedures thoroughly before making contact with a respondent. The interviewer should have all supplemental materials, such as introductory and fallback statements and visual aids, organized in advance for easy access. The interviewer should always be wearing his or her identification badge and should carry any other documentation, including informed consent forms required for the particular project. If the interview is to be done using CAPI, the interviewer needs to make sure the equipment is functional and that the laptop battery is charged.

Beginning the Interaction/Dealing With Refusals

This part of the manual emphasizes the need for the interviewer to be professional, both in what he or she says and in personal appearance. (This does not mean the interviewer needs to show up for interviews in a power suit. Interviewer dress should take into consideration what may be appropriate for the target population and the location of the interview.) The interviewer is reminded to memorize the introductory script and to state his or her name and the name of the sponsoring organization immediately upon meeting a respondent or potential respondent.

This part of the manual emphasizes that the initial stage of the interview conversation is about gaining cooperation. Even when initial agreement has been obtained in advance, either by the interviewer or a specially trained recruiter, the interviewer still needs to establish good rapport with the respondent during the conversation that precedes the beginning of questioning. The interviewer can gain the respondent's cooperation by convincing him or her that the survey is important and worthwhile. A professional and friendly manner, a well-delivered introductory statement, and successful answers to respondent questions will help to ensure that the respondent feels comfortable proceeding with the interview.

A discussion of the importance of the interviewer's own state of mind is appropriate here. A confident manner builds trust and credibility. The interviewer's personal conviction that the survey is worthwhile can help motivate the respondent to participate. This part of the manual should include a reminder to the interviewer that success in engaging respondent interest at this point will minimize refusals, thus improving the chances that the survey will collect unbiased data, because more of the people initially chosen to participate will contribute their views. Suggested responses for dealing with refusal attempts (**refusal conversion**), such as those in Example 6.3, should be included in this part of the manual. Refusals can come at the time of a precall or at the time of a "cold" field visit (a visit that has not been previously arranged). Even if a respondent has initially agreed to be interviewed, he or she may attempt to avoid going through with the survey when the interviewer arrives for the scheduled appointment. Recruiters and interviewers need to be well prepared with polite responses to such attempts; such responses may convince many respondents to reconsider.

EXAMPLE 6.3

Possible Responses to Refusal Attempts

Too busy   This should only take a few minutes. Sorry to have caught you at a bad time. I would be happy to call back. When would be a good time to call in the next day or two?

Bad health   I'm sorry to hear that. I would be happy to call back in a day or two. Would that be okay?

Too old   The opinions of older people are just as important in this survey as anyone else's. For the results to be representative, we have to be sure that older people have as much chance to give their opinion as anyone else does. We really want your opinion.

Feel inadequate   The questions are not at all difficult. There are no right or wrong answers. We are concerned about how you feel rather than how much you know about certain things. Some of the people we have already interviewed had the same concern you have, but once we got started, they didn't have any difficulty answering the questions. Maybe I could read just a few questions to you so you can see what they are like.

Not interested   It's very important that we get the opinions of everyone in the sample. Otherwise, the results won't be very useful. So I'd really like to talk with you.

No one's business   I can certainly understand. That's why all of our interviews are confidential. Protecting people's privacy is one of our major concerns, so we do not put people's names on the interview forms. All the results are reported in such a way that no individual can be linked with any answer.

Example 6.3 continued

Object to surveys   The questions in this survey are ones that [the survey organization] really needs answers to, and we think your opinions are important.

Don't allow strangers into home   Yes, I understand your reluctance to let strangers into your home. There are things we can do in order to make you feel more comfortable. For example, you can have a family member or friend in the house during the interview, or we can do the interview in some other location, like a library, a hotel lobby, or a neighbor's house. Or you could come to our survey office in [location]. We would be glad to reimburse you for your transportation costs.

The manual should also instruct the interviewer that it is best to terminate the conversation politely and leave the door open for a future attempt if an individual remains reluctant to participate after the interviewer has made an initial persuasion attempt. Sometimes it is better simply to try again on another day with a different approach, or perhaps a different interviewer should try. The manual should state clearly that every interviewer runs into respondents who refuse, but that, with experience, an interviewer's personal refusal rate will usually decrease. It is important that interviewers know and accept the fact that a few people will simply be unwilling to participate.

Establishing the Environment

Happily, most respondents do agree to interviews. The manual should describe the possible environments for interviews (in respondents' homes, the survey office, public locations, and so on) and provide the interviewer with a protocol for things to keep in mind in setting up a space for the interview. Certain details will depend on the population being interviewed and the subject of the survey. For example, older individuals being interviewed about health issues may need to be asked to bring their medication bottles and their glasses with them to the interview. In the interest of privacy and minimal distractions, the interviewer should be instructed to avoid an audience, but to do so as politely as possible. Example 6.4 lists some tactful ways in which interviewers might seek to gain privacy for themselves and their respondents.

EXAMPLE 6.4
Tactful Approaches to Establishing Privacy

- "If your friend would excuse us, maybe we could go into another room."

- "Many people prefer to answer the questions privately. Would it be okay to set up at the table in the kitchen (since other family members are busy in the living room)?"

- "Could we go into another room so we don't interfere with your family's activities?"

- *If at a survey office*: "We can do the interview in our interview room while your family waits here in the lobby, or they can pick you up in half an hour if that's more convenient."

- *If meeting in a hotel lobby:* "Perhaps your daughter would enjoy doing some browsing in the hotel stores while we find a spot away from the lobby noise to do the interview."

If the study specifically permits the presence of another person (for example, with older respondents who have cognitive difficulties, sometimes interviews are not possible without the assistance of family members), this part of the manual should tell the interviewer exactly what level of involvement is permissible and how to document the presence of another person in the interview. Usually, the third person present is asked not to answer for the respondent but may be allowed to repeat questions for the respondent and/or repeat answers for the interviewer. Sometimes the helper is simply there for emotional support.

Survey researchers know, however, that the mere presence of a third party during an interview (even if he or she says nothing) can influence how the respondent answers questions. The interview may touch on issues the respondent would not mind talking about with a stranger, but would prefer not to discuss with a loved one. The surveyor needs to weigh the potential loss of an entire interview (if a respondent is not able or willing to do the interview alone) against possible inaccurate answers to some items if a support person is allowed to be present. It is important that interviewers be instructed to code in the interview or on a face sheet whether another person was present during an interview, so that interviews done with and without another person present can be compared later for any consistent differences in response patterns.

This part of the manual should also instruct the interviewer about how to arrange suitable seating for the interview. In general, interviewers and respondents should be close enough to establish eye contact and to be able to hear each other. People of different cultures are comfortable with different amounts of interpersonal distance, so these instructions should take into consideration the cultural context of the survey. If there are no special cultural needs for more or less distance, the usual recommendation of 3 feet between interviewer and respondent is probably appropriate.

This part of the manual may also include information for the interviewer regarding the importance of obtaining informed consent, and should give instructions for presenting the form, having the respondent sign it, and providing the respondent with a copy before the questioning begins.

A final and important point about the interview environment is the safety of the interviewer. If interviews are done in respondents' homes or other public locations, there is always a concern that an interviewer could end up in an unfamiliar neighborhood or in a household where he or she might not feel safe. Interviewers should be encouraged to follow their instincts. The manual should instruct them that if they ever feel unsafe, they should simply take their leave, even if it means breaking off an interview before it is complete. Interviewers should carry cell phones so that they can call for help if necessary, and they should be reminded to keep the phones charged. The manual should tell interviewers explicitly that they must always let a supervisor know where they will be and for how long. If possible, it might be wise for interviewers to travel to designated interview locations in pairs, or a supervisor might accompany an interviewer.

Asking the Questions

This part of the interviewer training manual explains the importance of maintaining a neutral manner when conducting interviews. A neutral manner is one that does not imply criticism, surprise, approval, or disapproval of anything the respondent says, or of anything contained in the questionnaire. The point is that the interviewer must refrain from any behaviors that could influence how the respondent answers the questions. The manual should emphasize the concept of standardization—that is, the importance of asking all questions in the order presented and exactly as worded. It should be explained to the interviewer that the less variation there is in the way interview questions are delivered from one interview to another and from one interviewer to another, the better the chances are that answers will be comparable across respondents. All respondents need to hear the same questions to ensure the comparability of their answers.

The manual should tell the interviewer not to read response categories aloud unless they are part of the question or the questionnaire instructs the interviewer to read them. During questionnaire preparation, thought was given to whether or not response options should be offered the respondent, depending on the nature of the question. It is the interviewer's job to make sure that the decisions made in question preparation are carried out, to maximize data quality.

This part of the manual also explains the use of prompts if they are included in the questionnaire. Prompts are scripted statements that the interviewer is instructed to use when the respondent seems confused or unclear about how to answer a question. For example, when asked how many cigarettes he or she smokes in a day, a hesitant respondent might be prompted with "A pack contains 20 cigarettes." Prompts are printed on the questionnaire near the items they support, set off in some way (e.g., in boldface type or enclosed in boxes) so that the interviewer knows he or she should read them only if needed. The interviewer should be reminded that prompts should always be read verbatim from the questionnaire.

Probing

Probing is a technique for obtaining more information if a respondent gives an answer that is unclear, irrelevant, or incomplete. Probes may be verbal or nonverbal. This part of the manual should remind the interviewer of the importance of keeping probes neutral; examples such as those listed in Example 6.5 should be provided. Examples of poor probes—that is, probes that interviewers should not employ because they make interpretations—are also useful (see Example 6.6).

EXAMPLE 6.5
Proper Interview Probes

Show interest. An expression of interest and understanding, such as "uh-huh," "I see," and "yes," conveys the message that the response has been heard and more is expected.

Pause. Silence can tell a respondent that you are waiting to hear more.

Repeat the question. This can help a respondent who has not understood or misinterpreted the question or who has strayed from the question to get back on track. A neutral preface before repeating a question can help you to avoid sounding too mechanical:

"Yes, but . . ."
"Can you tell me overall . . ."
"But in general . . ."
"But in the country as a whole . . ."
"No one knows for sure, but . . ."
"We're just interested in your opinion . . ."

Repeat part of the question. You can, for example, repeat the frame of reference.

Repeat the reply. This can stimulate the respondent to say more, or to recognize an inaccuracy.

Ask a neutral question. Neutral questions can focus the respondent without biasing the response. Some examples:

For clarification:
"What do you mean exactly?"
"Could you please explain that?"

Example 6.5 continued

For specificity:
    "Could you be more specific about that?"
    "Tell me about that. What, who, how, why?"
    "Which would be closer?"
    (repeat response options)
        "So would you say that is . . . ?
    (repeat response options)

For relevance:
    "I see. Well, let me ask you again"
    (REPEAT QUESTION AS WRITTEN).
    "Would you tell me how you mean that?"

For completeness:
    "What else?"
    "Can you think of an example?"

For "don't know" answers:
    "You can take a minute to think about it."
    "Can you give me your best estimate?"

SOURCE: Adapted from the Kaiser/UCLA Sigmoid Study and Center for Health Studies, Group Health Cooperative.

EXAMPLE 6.6

Improper Probing

Question: "About how many hours of television would you say you watch in a 24-hour period?"

Answer: "Oh, I watch TV all day."

Improper probe: "So you mean about 12 hours?"

Better probe: "Could you be more specific? About how

many *hours* of television would you say you watch in a 24-hour period?"

Comment: The improper probe puts words in the respondent's mouth. It is better to make a polite request for a more specific answer and then repeat the question, emphasizing the need for an answer in *hours*, without making any assumptions.

Clarifying

When a respondent doesn't understand a word or a question, he or she may ask the interviewer for clarification. This part of the manual should let interviewers know that they will be given a document that lays out the specific clarifications they may give to respondents in such cases. This document is called the **question-by-question specifications** (or Q by Qs); it is also sometimes referred to as the *item-by-item rationale.* The Q by Qs contain all of the clarifications interviewers may give; they should be instructed not to give any others. If the clarifications in the Q by Qs do not help the respondent, the interviewer should be trained to refer the respondent back to his or her own interpretations with comments such as "Whatever that means to you" or "I'm afraid I'm not supposed to give you my own opinions. Could you just interpret it however seems best to you?"

Sometimes, a respondent may understand the questions but find it frustrating to have to answer several similar-sounding questions, or may find the topics, wording, or even the ordering of some questions to be objectionable. Such a respondent may ask the interviewer about the logic of preparing the questionnaire in a such a way. If the questionnaire has been carefully constructed, there usually are reasons for the particular order of questions or the repetitiveness the respondent perceives (see Chapter 3), but these reasons can be difficult to discuss in the interview setting and may be beyond the interviewer's level of training.

The interviewer can respond with polite statements such as the following: "We may have talked about this before, but they want me to ask each question as it is written"; "We may have touched on this in a previous question, but let me read this one just to be sure I've got your response correctly"; "I know it may be a little hard to understand why, but they want me to ask it in this way"; or "I'm not sure I can explain the reason, but they trained me to ask it in this way."

Sometimes the respondent is the one who needs to provide clarification. The interviewer may not be able to keep up with the respondent when attempting to record a lengthy or confusing text response verbatim, or the respondent may give an answer that seems to contradict a previous answer. The interviewer can ask for clarification with comments like "Let me be sure I've got this all down" or "Let me be sure I've got this right," and then repeating the answer. If an answer seems to contradict a previous response, the interviewer can say, "I may have misunderstood you" or "I may have made a mistake on a previous question. Let me just repeat the question and the response I thought you gave to see if this is right." When further details are needed, the interviewer can use the probes for clarification shown in Example 6.5.

Reinforcing the Respondent

This part of the manual is aimed at helping the interviewer help the respondent. Interviewers receive thorough training and practice in how to be interviewers, but respondents don't get the same kind of instruction about how to be respondents. There may be an unconscious expectation that respondents will intuitively know how to fit their thoughts into predetermined response choices or will answer the questions that are asked rather than questions they would prefer to talk about. Respondents may find it appropriate and pleasant to digress and ramble in the course of what they may consider to be an interesting conversation. Through neutral probing and clarifying, the interviewer can help guide the respondent to answer meaningfully. In addition, by using neutral positive reinforcement, interviewers can help respondents get the hang of the interview process. Using such reinforcement only when respondents provide clear, complete, and relevant answers can help focus respondents on the interview process. Neutral phrases that interviewers can use to reinforce respondents include "Thanks," "That's helpful," That's useful information," and "We appreciate getting your opinion on that."

Closing the Interaction

This part of the manual addresses how the interviewer can best end the interview session. The interviewer should be reminded of the importance of thanking each respondent and acknowledging the important role he or she has played by participating in the interview. The interviewer may spend some time at this point answering questions the respondent may have and discussing concerns that may have come up regarding the content of the survey. In fact, depending on the content of the questionnaire, a short "debriefing" conversation may be a positive way to end the interview. The interview questions may have raised some emotional concerns for the respondent. For example, parents who have been questioned about their children's exposure to potentially toxic substances may have become fearful that their children are at risk for serious health problems. They may need to be reassured that no causative links between studied exposures and specific diseases are yet known to exist and that none may be found. The interviewer could refer the respondent to a source of any information on what *is* known at this time, if appropriate. Many survey researchers whose studies deal with sensitive subjects often provide resources to respondents at the end of interviews. If the topic of the interview is domestic violence, for example, a list of shelters, hot lines, and counseling services may be provided in case the interview sparks a desire for more information or assistance.

THE INTERVIEWER'S RESPONSIBILITIES

This section of the interviewer training manual tells the interviewer what he or she is expected to know and do. The individual responsibilities are spelled out in the sections discussed below.

Contacting Respondents

This part of the manual gives the interviewer detailed instructions regarding how respondents are to be contacted. If interviews will be conducted "cold" in the field after households are chosen according to a sampling procedure, the procedure should be described in detail. If there is some other sampling procedure, every step should be spelled out, and trainers should make sure that the interviewers understand it well enough to implement it in the field. If advance contact is to be made, the manual should tell the interviewer how to go about it. For example, if the interviewers need to make appointments with respondents by telephone, the manual should describe when the interviewers are to make the calls (days of the week and times of day); how the interviewers will know what telephone numbers to call; what they should do in the case of no answers, busy signals, answering machines, wrong numbers, and unavailable respondents; and how to record call attempts. In-person interviewers should also be told what they should do if no one is at home when they knock on a door—for example, how many times to return to the same household and whether to call to reschedule an appointment ("stopping by" on the weekend to catch a respondent who previously agreed to an interview and then failed to be home at the appointed time is another option). The manual should include detailed information on the survey study's internal procedures for tracking contact attempts.

Also in this part of the training manual, interviewers should be told how interviews will be labeled for identification (usually using a numbering system) and how they are to record the outcome status of each interview. A copy of the form the surveyor has prepared for the interviewer to use in recording the outcome of each interview should be included in the manual; such forms usually include places for the interviewer to fill in the time and date of the interview, its length, any problems encountered, and respondent questions that a supervisor might need to answer. The form might also have spaces where the interviewer can give his or her interpretation of the respondent's attitude toward surveys and any reasons why a refusal or termination partway through the interview took place.

The interviewer should be instructed regarding how to fill out all the necessary information on this form, which is separate from the questionnaire but matched to it by the interview identification number. This outcome form (or interview face sheet) is tracked separately from the interview itself. The survey team can use the outcome forms to help them determine whether all of the questionnaires administered in the field (whether on paper or in electronic form) have made it back to the survey center for processing. The survey project's supervisors can also use the outcome forms as the basis for determining interviewers' productivity, or the number of completed interviews compared to hours worked. Example 6.7 provides a sample of a typical interview summary form.

EXAMPLE 6.7
Sample Interview Summary Form

INTERVIEWER: Answer the following questions about the interview.

Interviewer   _____

Date   _____

Interview Start Time _____   End Time _____

Overtime   _____

Example 6.7 continued

Which of the following best describes the respondent's attitude?

Very antagonistic	1
Somewhat antagonistic	2
Neutral	3
Somewhat helpful	4
Very helpful	5

How would you describe the respondent's interest in the interview?

Very *un*interested	1
Somewhat *un*interested	2
Neutral	3
Somewhat interested	4
Very interested	5

Did the respondent ask any questions about the survey?

Yes	1
No	2
Specify: _____	

ANSWER THE FOLLOWING *ONLY* IF THIS WAS A REFUSAL OR PARTIAL COMPLETION.

When did the respondent end the interview? (Specify exact place—i.e., question number) _____

WHERE TERMINATED _____

Which best describes how the interview was terminated?

No warning or explanation	1
An explanation to which you were not given a chance to respond	2
An explanation to which you *were* able to respond	3

Example 6.7 continued

Please explain the exact situation under which the interview was terminated:

_____

_____

_____

_____

Interviewer: _____

(signature)

Received and edited by: _____

Validation: _____

This form, along with the completed interview, is turned in to the survey center. Paper interviews are either handed in or, if the study is large and has remote interviewing areas, sometimes copies are made at the interviewing sites and the original questionnaires are mailed to the survey center. Such procedures are becoming less common, however. In large studies and in those where interviews are conducted in remote areas, surveyors are more likely to choose the CAPI method. The use of computers in administering surveys allows interviewers to e-mail completed interviews to the survey center, submit them on diskette, or upload them via the Internet to a server at the survey center. If such procedures are to be used in a survey, the training manual needs to spell them out clearly, and trainers need to make sure that the interviewers understand them.

This part of the manual should also explain that, no matter how the completed questionnaire is returned to the survey center, once it arrives, a supervisor will edit it for completeness, clarity in the recording of responses, and status information. The interviewer should be made aware that it may be necessary for him or her to recontact the respondent to obtain responses to items that were either overlooked or answered unclearly.

Confidentiality

The training manual should cover the ethics of survey interviewing. It is extremely important that interviewers understand their ethical responsibility to maintain the **confidentiality** of the people interviewed. This means not only following protocol regarding not putting names on individual questionnaires but also conducting interviews in private settings and not sharing a person's responses with anyone. (If interviewers are instructed to upload completed questionnaires via the Internet, the survey researcher must take care that an encryption process is in place, to make sure information cannot be intercepted.)

This part of the manual should thoroughly review the statements of confidentiality prepared for the introductory remarks of the interview as well as any internal procedures that are in place to protect respondents' privacy, such as keeping completed questionnaires in a locked cabinet. Interviewers should be reminded that "identifier" information, such as names, addresses, and telephone numbers, should never be contained within completed interviews. Such information must be recorded on separate cover sheets or in a log that links ID numbers to the correct information. If the interview was done in CAPI, identifier information should be in a separate electronic or paper file, not in the interview itself, so the identifiers are not transmitted to the survey center together with that person's data. Completed interviews should be stored in a secure location for a period of time following the survey until data entry is completed (if paper questionnaires are used) and the data files are cleaned of improper codes. The raw interviews can then be destroyed. Interviewers should be cautioned not to discuss any of the results during or after completion of the survey.

How to Use the Interview

This part of the manual outlines the conventions in the interview format, including standard abbreviations (e.g., typically, a question on the questionnaire is referred to as a Q, a respondent is an R, an informant who gives information about an R is referred to as an I, and DK indicates that the respondent said, "I don't know"). The interviewer will need repeated exposure to these conventions to become comfortable using them. Example 6.8 presents a list of possible questionnaire conventions.

EXAMPLE 6.8
Sample Interview Format Conventions

- Instructions to the interviewer are in CAPS.

- Capitalized portions are not read to the respondent.

- Skip patterns are identified using arrows followed by the number of the Q you should move to next.

- Prompts are printed in boldface and set off to the right of the Q. Read them exactly as printed if R seems unclear about answering the Q.

- Standard prompts are not printed on the questionnaire but may be used for any Q unless you are instructed not to use prompts in the Q by Qs for that item. Refer to the list of standard prompts in your interviewer manual.

This part of the manual should also tell the interviewer how to record information and how to indicate any corrections, whether the survey is being conducted on paper or using CAPI (see Examples 6.9, 6.10, and 6.11).

EXAMPLE 6.9
Sample Instructions for Recording Information on the Paper Questionnaire

- Write clearly, neatly, and legibly.

- Write "DK" when the respondent does not know the answer to a question.

- If you used a probe to get more information on a question, write an "X" in the margin. For multiple probes, write that number of Xs.

- To record answers to precoded questions, circle the number of the response given.

- Answers to open-ended questions must be written verbatim. Do not paraphrase.

EXAMPLE 6.10
Sample Instructions for Recording Information in CAPI

- Make your entries accurately.

- Type the number of the response given by R for precoded items.

- Press enter to display the next applicable question.

- If multiple choices are possible, CAI will allow you to mark all choices before pressing enter. If only one choice is allowed, CAI will prevent you from making multiple entries for one question.

- You can make a text note anywhere in the interview for clarification of a response. Press F1 and a text

Example 6.10 continued

pad will appear on the screen. Make a careful text entry and press enter to close the text box and continue questioning.

- If you use standard probes, type F1 and mark an X for every probe in the text box.

- If you are ever in doubt about how to code a response, write the answer out verbatim in the text pad (F1).

Comment: These instructions apply only to this particular CAPI survey; CAI programs vary, so instructions to interviewers about how to use them will vary also.

EXAMPLE 6.11
Sample Instructions for
Making Corrections in the Interview

On Paper:

If you mark the wrong answer choice, or R changes his/her mind after the response has been marked, make a single diagonal line through the incorrect answer and mark the correct one. Write IE by the crossed-out response if it was an interviewer error, or write RE if it was a respondent-initiated change, or respondent error.

In CAPI:

The CAI software used for this project is programmed not to allow you simply to change an incorrect response choice. This forces you to document all corrections. Open the text pad and type IE for interviewer error or RE for respondent error if the respondent changed his/her mind. Then type in what the correct answer should have been, as well as any notes (F1) to clarify the entry.

Special Procedures

If there are any sections of the questionnaire that require special training, they should be addressed in this section of the manual, and trainers should be sure to cover this material in the training sessions. For example, health research survey projects sometimes require interviewers to administer standardized screening measures to determine whether respondents may have particular types of problems, such as depression, alcohol dependence, or cognitive impairment. Interviewers must clearly understand that they are not expected to diagnose respondents in the way a clinician would. This part of the training manual should include explicit instructions on how such screening measures are to be administered, and interviewers should be trained regarding how they are to respond to unexpected situations. Interviewers' fears regarding such special procedures should be addressed in training, and interviewers should be told how they can obtain help (such as immediate contact with a supervisor or responsible clinician) if difficult circumstances arise.

Use of Technology

The training manual should also provide detailed instructions regarding any interview procedures involving technology, and interviewers should have the opportunity to practice these procedures in training. This part of the manual should include instructions for the use of any CAI software, and interviewers should be given hands-on computer training. Some interviewers who are used to working with paper questionnaires need to get used to seeing only small portions of the interview on the screen at a time. Instructions should include how to open a new interview versus a completed interview that is being edited, and interviewers should be reminded of the importance of correctly entering identifiers such as ID number and date of interview. Example 6.12 shows a sample of a screen in a CAPI questionnaire.

EXAMPLE 6.12
Sample CAPI Screen

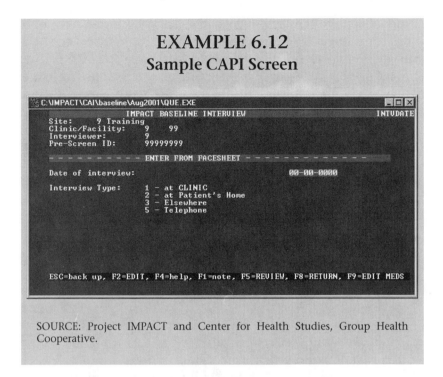

SOURCE: Project IMPACT and Center for Health Studies, Group Health Cooperative.

To instruct interviewers in the use of computers for interviewing, the trainer may need to bring a number of extension cords into a conference room so that an individual laptop can be plugged in for each trainee. The trainer can project each question from a laptop onto a large screen as the trainees work through the questionnaire and practice recording and correcting responses. If there are special procedures for routing interviews once they are completed, the trainer should have the interviewers practice these as well. The trainer should also walk the trainees through the steps of backing up each set of interviews (that is, making and storing electronic copies), archiving the backup copies (that is, saving them in a computer file), and any Internet uploading or downloading procedures they will need to use. As noted above, in large studies, interviewers may be asked to send completed interviews to the survey center as e-mail attachments or upload them via a Web site to a server at the survey center, rather than dealing with diskettes. Uploading procedures, although not difficult, are fairly cutting edge. The procedures differ from study to study, as they are designed by programmers to suit particular projects' needs. The procedures may seem foreign to trainees; they should be spelled out clearly in the training manual, and the trainees should have plenty of opportunities to practice them. Example 6.13 presents a sample set of uploading instructions for interviewers.

EXAMPLE 6.13
Sample Instructions for Uploading Completed Interview Files to a Web Site

You will be given a log-on ID for the project Web site at www.survey.xxx. Once a week, you will upload your completed interviews to the Web site. Every time you do an interview, it will be saved in a file. The file name ends with .dat. This is the file you will upload weekly.

To upload via the Web:

1. Open your Internet browser.

2. Enter the following Internet address: http://www.survey.location.xxx.

3. Choose "Survey Information Systems" from the menu. The Web site with logo will be displayed, along with two boxes for user name and password.

4. Enter your user name and password and click "enter" on the screen (hitting the enter key on your keyboard will not work).

Example 6.13 continued

5. A menu bar will appear at the bottom of the screen. Click on "interviews."

6. On the next menu bar, choose "file transfer."

7. For security reasons, you will be asked for your user name and password again. Reenter them.

8. A screen will display showing a small window (called "upload file") with a browse button next to it. Click on "browse."

9. Your files will appear in a directory format. Click on the file you wish to upload. The name of the file will appear in the "upload file" box on the screen.

10. Click "upload" and your file will be sent to the server at the survey center.

SOURCE: Adapted from Project IMPACT.

Editing the Interview

Editing a completed questionnaire consists of looking it over to find and correct errors, clarify handwriting, and add clarifying notes. In this section of the training manual, interviewers should be told that they need to edit every questionnaire before turning it in and that a supervisor or other reviewer will do a second edit. Interviewers should also be informed that if errors or incomplete sections are found during a second edit, they will be asked to make corrections and possibly will be expected to call respondents back to fill in missing data. Interviewers should be encouraged to edit their questionnaires as soon after the completion of the interviews as possible. For example, if interviews are being done in respondents' homes, many interviewers will edit a just-completed questionnaire in the car before going on to the next respondent.

In CAPI, editing can be tricky, as some CAI programs make scrolling back and forth difficult. If the survey uses CAPI, this part of the manual should outline the process of moving through the computerized questionnaire for editing. Interviewers should be given clear instructions regarding all of the procedures for CAI, such as those in Example 6.14; these should include information about any quirks of the interview program. The trainer should make sure the interviewers have time to practice editing some questionnaires.

EXAMPLE 6.14
Sample CAI Instructions

Getting into the program	Go to current month's folder in Explorer. Double click on que.exe.
Starting the program	You will see a screen that asks you what you want to do. **BEGIN A NEW INTERVIEW** Allows you to begin a new interview, or to enter an ID for a case that you may have called on before, but did not begin the interview. **RESTART AN INTERVIEW** Allows you to "restart" a case. This may happen for a number of reasons: • Your previous contact was not at a good time for R, and you needed to call back. • R becomes tired, or breaks off during the interview for any reason, but is willing to complete it. • You need to return to the medications section in the baseline interview after completing the rest of the interview.

Example 6.14 continued

Using restart	The restart function is now always accessible. You will leave the case only by using CTRL + End.
	When you restart the case, you will return to the screen where you hit CTRL + End. If you need to go back (for instance, if you are in the contact script), you may hit Esc to do so to get to the correct script item.
	DO NOT go back beyond Item: Contact and then hit CTRL + End. If you use this function at the face sheet input screen before Item: Contact, when you attempt to reenter the case, you will be told you have a duplicate ID. Then, when you exit the case, you will get a warning that says your data are not saved. This is true—your input from that contact will not be saved, as the system believes you were using a duplicate ID.
	Every time you override to input a duplicate ID, you create a file that "hides" behind the main ID file. This means that those people who pull the data off the Web site have to sort out the "supplemental" case IDs, which takes a lot of time. Please observe the rule in Number 3, above.
Entering the case ID	You will need to enter the case ID a total of three times: twice before you proceed to the initial face sheet entry screen, and another time after you complete the interviewer observations. This forces you to double-check the entry of IDs in the event you make an entry error.

Example 6.14 continued

Hot keys	F1 brings up a text field so that you may enter comments. This works at any screen. F4 = HELP. The help may consist of general Ci3 help, or a QxQ or recommended response for selected items F5 brings up the REVIEW function. This function enables you to select the item you need to review for editing, because you need to change a response at a previous item, etc. F8 brings up the RETURN function. This enables you to return to the last answered item. This function also checks logic, so if R changed an answer that affects the logical path (skips), you will go to the first omitted item. When all omitted items are completed, using this same hot key allows you to return to the first blank item. If this item is a dependent Q, you must return to the last substantive Q (main numbered item). F9 is a shortcut to "EDIT MEDS." This key is normally used in an interview that has been restarted just to complete entry of medications. After entering the ID number, you may press F9 to go directly to question Q49 and add (additional) medications not documented in the initial interview.
Text field	Use F1 to get it; hit enter twice to leave it.
Going back one or two screens	Use the Esc key to go back only one or two items.

Example 6.14 continued

Ending an interview when only partway through	Hit CTRL + End. Your computer will pause briefly while the data writes, and you will return to the initial entry screen.
Editing the interview	You will only use the CTRL + End function to exit a case. This will save you from getting a duplicate ID warning (see above for exception). You will return to edit as a "restart." Do your editing using your hot keys.

SOURCE: Project IMPACT and Center for Health Studies, Group Health Cooperative.

This part of the manual should also tell the interviewer how to record the status of the questionnaire in the process from interview completion through data entry. Many times, questionnaires are tracked using separate control sheets or face sheets that are attached or incorporated into the questionnaire cover sheets. When a task is completed, the date of completion is recorded on the control sheet, and the questionnaire is routed to the next step.

Example 6.15 illustrates a possible layout for a control sheet. Once the interview is complete and the interviewer has edited it, the interviewer dates and signs the form where indicated. When a reviewer has finished editing the questionnaire, he or she enters the date on the form and signs it on the "edit complete" line, and the questionnaire is routed back to the interviewer for corrections and callbacks, if necessary. On completion of corrections, the interviewer signs the form again and routes the questionnaire to data entry. Once data are entered, the questionnaire may be filed.

If the interview was done using CAPI, an electronic copy should have been kept on the interviewer's computer at the

EXAMPLE 6.15
Sample Control Sheet

STATUS   DATE   SIGNATURE

Interview Complete   _____   _____

Edit Complete   _____   _____

Corrections Complete   _____   _____

Data Entry Complete (if paper)/
Electronic Received (if CAPI)_____   →FILE

time the interview was submitted to the reviewer for editing. The interviewer would then correct this version and resubmit the corrected questionnaire by whatever mechanism is being used (e-mail attachment, diskette, or upload to a server). The survey center may also choose to limit possible confusion over which version of the interview is newest by making the corrections centrally, directly in the database containing the submitted interview, in communication with the interviewer. It is very important that interviewers understand how to document changes and keep track of dates that corrections are made, so that the survey team can be sure which version of an interview is the most up-to-date. Once corrections are made, any copies of the older version should be deleted from the main database, but these may be labeled and stored in a "history" file in case questions arise later.

APPENDICES

Question-by-Question Specifications for Interview Questions

The Q by Qs for the interview questions should be compiled into a detailed document and included in the interviewer training manual as an appendix. The Q by Qs should inform the interviewer about the purpose of each item and should provide any special instructions for how to ask it, probe it, or record foreseeable answers that may not intuitively fit an answer category. Understanding the rationale behind the inclusion of individual items can help the interviewer to recognize whether a response has actually answered a question in a useful way or needs a probe. Example 6.16 shows some samples of Q by Qs.

EXAMPLE 6.16
Sample Specifications for Interview Questions

Question: What is your current marital status?

Explanation: We are interested in the respondent's current (meaning most recent) marital status. Those people who live with someone other than a spouse will be picked up in Question 5 (Do you live with other family members or with someone else?).

Question: Think about the walking you typically do each day. On average, how many miles do you walk each day? Count the distance you walk for exercise, to work, as part of your job, to the bus, to the store, and so on. Don't try to estimate the distance you walk while inside your home or office.

_____ miles OR _____ blocks

Prompt: **A mile is equal to 12 city blocks.**

Explanation: The intent of this question is to estimate any active walking the respondent may do during the course of a typical day. Do not ask the respondent to estimate incidental walking that may take place at home or at work, such as walking to the refrigerator to get water or moving from desk to filing cabinet.

Example 6.16 continued

Question: Have the medications you have taken in the past for depression been helpful?

Explanation: The purpose of the question is to determine whether and how much previous medication use has helped with depression symptoms. Read response categories in lowercase. If R reports one medication as very helpful but another as not helpful at all, ask R to answer for the one that helped (or helped the most) and record that response.

SOURCE: Adapted from the Kaiser/UCLA Sigmoid Study and Project IMPACT.

Sample Interview

It is helpful to include a paper copy of the actual interview questionnaire in the training manual, even if the interview will be done using CAPI. One drawback of CAPI is that the interviewer sees one question at a time, and so cannot get a sense of the big picture and flow of the entire instrument. The interviewer needs to study the "real thing" in its entirety before attempting to conduct practice interviews. If the questionnaire is not yet finished when the training manual is being prepared, the most recent draft should be included.

Forms and Administrative Procedures

Samples of forms such as the interview summary form (Example 6.7) and the interview control sheet (Example 6.15) should be included in the training manual so the interviewer can learn how to fill them out. By keeping track of interview contacts and outcomes, the surveyor gets a good idea of the level of response. These records also inform the supervisors of refusals that may have to be converted and return visits or callbacks that will have to be scheduled. It is best if the survey team can analyze the contact records every day to determine the progress of the survey, the response rate (which is calculated at the end of each interviewing day), and the productivity of interviewers, and to note any field problems that may arise.

In large surveys, someone should be assigned the specific task of monitoring the status of every interview and sample unit contact. This person would also be responsible for distributing new sample units. The contact record is very important to quality control in surveys. Example 6.17 shows how a contact record might be designed. Another form of documentation is the telephone screening log, which is used if contact is made by phone before in-person contact is made. Example 6.18 displays a sample of such a log.

Survey interviewers may also need to learn how to fill out other forms, such as time sheets for recording their hours worked and forms for reimbursement of any out-of-pocket expenses they may have related to their work (e.g., for telephone calls and mileage). Copies of these forms should also be included in the training manual.

SUPERVISION TO BE PROVIDED

Interviewers need to know not only what is expected of them, but what they may expect of the survey center and supervisory staff. Trainers should explain to interviewers how they may contact the center for questions and help with unexpected problems in the field. Any regular support that will be provided, such as regular staff meetings and/or conference calls, should be outlined, and interviewers should be told how they will be informed of any updates in procedures. It is also important that interviewers understand how their performance will be monitored and evaluated.

Interviewer training manuals vary from project to project and in accordance with the background knowledge of the trainees. Not every training manual will cover all of the topics described above. What should be included and in what

EXAMPLE 6.17
Sample Contact Record

Field/In-Person Contact Record

Period From: To:

Interviewer:

Date	Neighborhood Code	Interview Start Time	Interview End Time	Outcome

CI = Completed Interview   RF = Refusal
NH = Not Home   CB = Come Back

Mileage:
       Date: Miles:
1.
2.
3.
4.
5.

Interviewer Signature: Total Hours:
Supervisor Signature: Total Miles:

Example 6.17 continued

Comment: This form may be used to document contact attempts in the field and how they turned out (e.g., respondent not home versus interview completed) and the amount of time each interview took. In this example, the surveyor has chosen to include a mileage record on the same form for travel reimbursement purposes.

EXAMPLE 6.18
Sample Telephone Screening Log

Respondent Name: _____

Screening ID#: __ __ __ - __ __ __ __

Phone Number: _____

Address: _____

_____

Attempt #	Date	Day of Week	Time of Day	Caller	Outcome Code/Notes

OUTCOME CODES:

CI = Completed Interview   BZ = Busy Signal

RF = Refusal   AM = Answering Machine

NA = No Answer   DS = Disconnected

CB = Call Back   WN = Wrong Number

Example 6.18 continued

Comment: A form like this may be used to keep track of all call attempts for a particular possible respondent being contacted for either screening or recruitment.

order will depend on the survey, the experience levels of the interviewers being trained, and the trainers' preferences. No matter what is included, however, the language in the manual should be direct. Complex topics, such as sampling, need not be described in scientific detail. Brief remarks to give context, followed by the steps the interviewer must follow, should suffice. Example 6.19 presents some excerpts from a sample training manual for in-person interviewers. In addition to the content described above and that illustrated in Example 6.19, the training manual might include a summary list of behaviors that interviewers should avoid, as in Example 6.20.

EXAMPLE 6.19
Excerpts From a Sample Training Manual
for In-Person Interviewers

Description of the Survey

This project will test a questionnaire designed to identify older persons who may be at risk for developing
health problems from alcohol use. The questionnaire
will be used to search for people who are not yet known
to be at risk so they can be educated before problems
occur. Although a number of questionnaires already
exist that can identify people at risk for alcohol dependence and abuse, none is currently available to find people at risk for problems from drinking *small* amounts of
alcohol, especially among the elderly. Such problems
include depression, intensified effects of alcohol due to
certain illnesses or medications (leading to injuries), and
ineffective treatment of chronic conditions such as dia-
betes due to alcohol use. The ultimate purpose of the
new survey is to help identify persons at risk for such
problems so they can be helped to avoid them.

The survey was constructed with input from many
experts in several fields of study. The questions were
very thoughtfully chosen and should logically be able to
find the persons who are at risk. However, we do not yet
know if the survey actually works in identifying the
"right" people. You are entering the project at a very
important point: the testing process to see if the survey
works. This is called a *validation test.* When a question or
questionnaire is valid, that means it measures what it is
intended to measure. You are going to help us find out if
the survey is a valid tool for identifying alcohol-related
problems.

Example 6.19 continued

Background on Survey Methods

Every research study has a *study design* that was developed to answer *research questions*. The primary research question for this project is "Does the survey reliably identify older persons at risk for alcohol-related problems?" A subquestion is "Can the survey be implemented usefully in senior-specific settings such as senior centers and retirement homes?" The study design thus involves having older persons complete questionnaires in these types of settings to find out how the survey performs. Respondents' answers are analyzed in a variety of ways to answer the research questions. Our current purpose is to make sure that the data collected from respondents are of high quality so that analysis will be meaningful.

A study design usually includes the following important components: sampling, data collection, and analysis.

Sampling: Sampling is the procedure by which survey participants (or *respondents*) are chosen. A sample is a subset of the entire group or *population* targeted by the survey. Because we cannot administer a questionnaire to every person in the county who is 65 years of age or older and drinks, we select a smaller group to *represent* the population. This group is our sample. As long as the smaller group is not different from the population in some significant way (e.g., we sample only females, or only people who wear glasses), we should be able to make predictions about how the survey will perform in the population in general.

There are many methods of sampling. The method chosen for this project is the *convenience* sample. The sample is "convenient" because we do not identify eligible people in advance by a scientific method that makes

Example 6.19 continued

sure *all* eligible persons have a chance to be included. We simply go to places where individuals in the appropriate age group may congregate and screen for eligible candidates. However, this sampling strategy is not convenient in many other ways. We cannot choose only the people who are easiest to approach, because we could be systematically excluding specific groups of people who might perform differently on the survey, such as more frail individuals. We will approach individuals in the dining areas and lobbies of the chosen sites. We must follow protocol carefully to make sure everyone who is eligible gets a chance to participate. We must also do our best to ensure a high *response rate.* The response rate is the number of eligible individuals who are actually interviewed. To maximize the response rate, we need to minimize the *refusal rate.* We will practice reasonable ways of persuading reluctant respondents to participate in an interview; however, we will not attempt to force them to participate. Our informed consent form says that participation is voluntary, and we must abide by that. Our ideal total *sample size* is 1,000 participants across sites. We expect to spend 10-12 months recruiting participants.

Data collection: Data collection is the process by which information is gathered and prepared for analysis. In this study, data collection consists of a series of protocols and procedures to administer the survey interview and keep track of the sample (i.e., numbers of men and women, drinkers and nondrinkers, refusers and ineligibles, and so on). Following these procedures carefully will help ensure usable, meaningful data from which to draw conclusions. The primary *data collection tool* for this study is a questionnaire administered by interview on a laptop computer.

Example 6.19 continued

You must maintain a neutral presence in your role as "data collector." Although it is an asset to be personable and friendly in your interactions with respondents, you are not there to help them decide how to answer the survey questions or to counsel them on their health or drinking behavior. Doing so could bias the survey results and create problems with respondents or site staff.

Analysis: Analysis consists of a multitude of statistical tests done on the data by statistics experts using computers. In order for meaningful analyses to be carried out, the data entered into the computer must be accurate and complete. Part of your job is to ensure that the data are as accurate and complete as possible for this step of the process. Warning: This does not mean that you should help respondents answer questions by interpreting meanings for them (except when instructed to do so on the screen). If you do that, we actually *lose* information because we do not find out that the question was confusing.

In order to be entered into the computer in a meaningful way, the data need to be *coded*. Coding involves translating a wordy response into a number or letter that represents the response in a way the computer can understand. Most of the questionnaire is *precoded;* you select the response given by the respondent by typing in the numeric code assigned to it on the screen. A few items on the survey require that you (the interviewer) fill in a code at the end of the interview.

Your Role

You have a role in each of the study components listed above. When you select people to approach in the lobby or lunchroom without excluding anyone inappropriately, you are helping to ensure as representative a

Example 6.19 continued

sample as possible. When you administer the interview
and fill out the contact forms (forms for documenting
how many people were approached, their eligibility status, and whether they chose to participate), you are performing data collection. And when you take care to
review forms and interviews for clarity and completeness before turning them in to the survey center, you are
helping to ensure meaningful analysis. You are very
important!

The Survey Center's Role

The survey center is responsible for supporting your
efforts in collecting accurate data, and for collecting and
processing the data. We will compare your contact
sheets to the interviews you submit to make sure there
are no missing interviews. Once a week, we will let you
know if there seems to be anything missing. If so, you
will be asked to look for and submit the information by
the end of the week. We will also edit each interview you
submit and give you written feedback about any errors,
so that you can avoid the same mistakes in the future.
Everyone makes mistakes, and we understand that interviews will never be perfect. But we will do our best to
give you constructive and timely feedback so you can do
your job well. We will also monitor the number of interviews you are able to complete per hour of work as well
as your response rate. We understand that these may
vary a great deal depending on which site you are working in at a given time. We are interested in quality more
than quantity. We will work with you to develop skills
that will help you to keep up productivity without com-
promising quality.

There will also be a weekly interviewer meeting during which you can get input from us as well as each

Example 6.19 continued

other on questions that have arisen for you during the week. Please feel free to raise anything that's on your mind. For quick troubleshooting assistance when you are in the field, call (999) 999-9999. For less urgent questions, please e-mail us at survey@problems.org.

Protocols and Procedures

As mentioned previously, protocols and procedures are subject to revision as we learn more about how to implement the study. Once the systems are in place, however, there should be little change. Following are the protocols and procedures as we have established them thus far.

The sampling protocol: Every lobby and cafeteria will have a different seating arrangement. The important thing is to work the room in a systematic way. Choose a logical starting point and approach every person who looks like he or she could be 50 years old or older. This is so that we do not miss anyone who is actually in the right age group (65 or older) but looks younger. Follow the recruitment script (below) to find out if the person is eligible, and, if appropriate, administer informed consent. Make arrangements to meet for the actual interview if the person consents. Move to the next person who looks to be 50 or older. Follow the seating pattern in the room until you reach the last chair. If new people have seated themselves while you were recruiting, simply start the pattern over, approaching only those people who are new.

The contact sheet: Recruiting people and administering the interview involves several steps that you should follow in order as much as possible. To help you keep track of the procedures, you will carry a checklist (on a clip-

Example 6.19 continued

board) with you at the site. Step 1 involves delivering the recruitment script and filling out a contact form. You basically find out if a person is eligible and willing to participate using the script, and record the outcomes on the form. Most of the sites will have flyers about the project posted in the room. You can refer to these in identifying yourself, or you may find that people ask you about the project because they have seen the flyer. If a person you have approached is eligible and willing, the next step is the informed consent. You must describe the form and get it signed before you can proceed.

The recruitment script/eligibility screen: The recruitment script is designed to help you find out quickly if someone is eligible to participate in the study. You need not be a parrot in delivering the script. Learn the content well enough to be able to say it conversationally. During the recruitment script, you will mention that there is a small gift as a token of thanks for the person's efforts in doing the interview. The script is in the appendix of this manual. The *eligibility criteria* for this study are as follows:

1. The person must be 65 years of age or older.

2. The person must have had at least 12 drinks of alcohol in any one year of his or her life, AND must have had at least one drink of alcohol in the past 12 months. Persons who have not had at least 12 drinks in any one year are ineligible.

3. The person must be able to understand English.

Example 6.19 continued

4. The person must *not* have participated in the study before.

The contact form: The contact form was designed to help us keep track not only of the characteristics of the people we include in the study, but also of those who are ineligible and those who refuse. A sample form appears in the appendix. Date, time, gender, ethnicity, age, drinking status, and outcome must be filled out for each person approached. If the person is ineligible or refuses to participate, the reason should be recorded. *Be sure to fill in your name, the site, and the page number on each page of the forms you use on a given day. Make notes of unusual situations.*

The informed consent form: Eligible persons who are willing to participate must give their informed consent in writing by signing the informed consent form. There is a form specific to each site that each respondent must read and sign. Please take time to review the consent form for your site, so you can be familiar with its contents. A script for describing the informed consent to people is in the appendix. Emphasize the confidential nature of the study.

The survey: The interview should be done at a time and place that is convenient for the respondent. You can make arrangements to meet in a small office each site will make available, perhaps even on the same day as screening, or you can go to the respondent's home or some other reasonable location. A paper copy of the most recent version of the interview is located in the rear pocket of this manual. Please review it, so you can become familiar with its contents.

Example 6.19 continued

Interviewing: Guidelines for conducting interviews are provided in the next chapter of this manual. We will practice interviewing skills in training. A separate manual is provided for CAPI training and practice.

The dementia screen: Because cognitive impairment can be a problem for older people, making interview responses difficult and possibly unreliable, we are using a short test; people who pass it are likely to be cognitively able to complete the interview. There will be a way to record the results of this screen on the contact sheet. To conduct the test, you read to the respondent a series of numbers, starting with two digits and increasing the number of digits by one each time until there are seven digits. You then ask the respondent to repeat each set of numbers and record exactly what he or she says on the contact sheet. You should read the numbers at a pace of about one digit per second; do not group the numbers (i.e., do not read with a longer pause after the first group of three, as you would for a phone number). Label the contact sheet and dementia screen materials with the ID number used for the interview.

Thank the person for participating and offer one of the incentives we will provide. There will be small gifts or a $5 payment offered for participation. The nature of the item may vary by site, or may be the choice of the participant.

SOURCE: Adapted from the Alcohol-Related Problems Survey Project (Arlene Fink Associates).

Comment: In these excerpts from a sample training manual, interviewers are first introduced to the specific project they will be working on; this is followed by general information about surveys and the steps involved in conducting them. Then interviewers are given specific

Example 6.19 continued

instructions in how to conduct the data collection, from sampling through distribution of the incentive. A great deal of detail is provided. Unusual components (such as the dementia screen) are specifically spelled out. The manual then has a second chapter (not shown) that goes into the details of interviewing skills, followed by an appendix containing forms, a copy of the interview, Q by Qs, and other pertinent materials. A separate manual is provided for CAPI training.

EXAMPLE 6.20
What Not to Do as an Interviewer

NEVER

Get involved in long explanations of the study
Try to explain sampling in detail
Deviate from the study introduction, sequence of questions, or question wording
Try to justify or defend what you are doing
Try to explain procedures or wording
Suggest an answer or agree or disagree with an answer
Interpret the meaning of a question
Try to ask questions from memory
Rush the respondent
Patronize the respondent
Dominate the interview
Let another person answer for the intended respondent
Interview someone you know
Falsify an interview
Improvise
Add response categories

Example 6.20 continued

Turn in a questionnaire without checking it over to be sure every question has been asked and its answer recorded

The Training Session

Although some surveys may not require more than a day of interviewer training, in general, interviewers are much better prepared if they have had 2 to 5 days of instruction and practice. Example 6.21 shows a sample agenda for interviewer training sessions. As the example illustrates, training usually begins with a review of the training manual that includes presentation and discussion. The most important part of training, however, centers on interviewing techniques, which are demonstrated by skilled presenters who also give expert feedback to trainees during role-playing. It cannot be emphasized enough that repeated practice, both in the training sessions and assigned as "homework," is essential for helping interviewers to develop excellent interviewing skills. In addition, if the interview is to be done using CAPI, it is crucial that interviewers become fluent in the use of the computer to administer the questionnaire. If field training is to be done, it can be scheduled during the classroom training period.

EXAMPLE 6.21
Agenda for Interviewer Training Sessions

DAY 1

Introductions
Review of the Training Manual
Description of the Survey

Example 6.21 continued

Protocols and Procedures
Introduction to Survey Methods
Interviewing Techniques and Guidelines
The Interviewer's Responsibilities
General Interview Demonstration

DAY 2

Review of Interviewer's Responsibilities and
    Interviewing Techniques
Question-by-Question Specifications
Use of the CAPI Instrument: Navigating on the Laptop
Practice Interviewing (Role-Playing)

DAY 3

More CAPI Role-Playing
Forms and Administrative Procedures
Getting Support From Supervisors and Fellow
    Interviewers
Wrap-Up and Practice Assignments
Field Training Scheduling

Supervision

Training is the beginning of equipping an interviewer to be a good collector of data. After training is completed, the maintenance of high-quality interviewing skills requires appropriate supervision. The surveyor must put in place some mechanism for monitoring interviewer performance; however, effective supervision is more than that. Supervision should be part of the implementation of a support structure to help build a sense of teamwork among interviewers to achieve a goal. Supervision of interviewers should include the following:

- Monitoring *interviewer performance* and providing constructive *feedback*

- Maintaining high levels of *standardization*

- Providing *interviewer support* that fosters a team spirit and pride in the quality of work done in the field

- Maintaining effective *communication* channels, both from supervisor to interviewer and vice versa

INTERVIEWER PERFORMANCE AND FEEDBACK

There are four main aspects of interviewer performance that require supervision: costs, response rates, the quality of the completed questionnaires, and the quality of the interviewing.

Costs

Interviewers can be "expensive" if they complete low numbers of interviews in relation to the amount of time they spend in the field. Interviewers might have low numbers of completed interviews if they are working at unproductive times, if they have high refusal rates (a refusal can take as much time as an interview), or if they are undisciplined in their work habits (e.g., they find other things to do). In the case of field interviewing, high mileage costs may be a problem if the interviewer lives far from the neighborhoods of the respondents. Supervisors need to look for such problems and give interviewers feedback. For instance, a supervisor might advise an interviewer about how to choose more productive times to work, or retrain an interviewer in the techniques for minimizing refusals.

Sometimes surveyors pay interviewers by the completed interview rather than by the hour to increase productivity, but they need to be aware that this can compromise quality if interviewers are tempted to rush to get more interviews done. When interviewers are paid by the interview, checks on the quality of the interviews completed are especially important.

Response Rates

The **response rate** in a sample is the degree to which cooperation is obtained from all eligible respondents. The rate at which persons agree to be interviewed is influenced by many factors, including sampling technique, the topic of the survey, and how appealing the survey sounds during the introduction. No particular rate is accepted as standard, but if rates of 70% to 80% are achieved, surveyors can feel comfortable with analyses based on the data. Survey researchers make every effort to achieve this rate for surveys of the general population; lower rates may be acceptable for specialized, homogeneous populations.

Response rates are subject to significant variation depending on how they are calculated. The correct rate is generally a reflection of how successful the survey team is in obtaining cooperation from the eligible respondents. It is the measure of the effectiveness of data collection and is determined as follows:

$$\text{Response rate} = \text{Number of completed} \\ \text{interviews} / \text{Number in sample eligible.}$$

Eligible respondents include those who complete interviews, those who are eligible but refuse to be interviewed, those who begin interviews but do not complete them, those who are eligible but not available for interview (e.g., due to illness), and those who are eligible but are not interviewed because a language barrier exists. Persons who are ineligible to be respondents are those who live in households where no member has the defining characteristics for inclusion, such as "adult over the age of 18" or "currently working full-time." Even if a household is never contacted, it is still considered eligible because there is no substantial evidence to eliminate it from the sampling pool.

When an interviewer has high refusal rates, a supervisor should investigate. If interviewers are assigned to different groups of potential respondents, higher refusal rates in one group may have nothing to do with the interviewer; the individuals in that group may be harder to enlist for some reason. However, some interviewers will have problems engaging respondents adequately to get their cooperation. Supervisors can retrain interviewers in delivering introductory remarks. Some interviewers may never get the hang of it, however, and may need to be taken off the project.

Supervisors sometimes assign interviewers who are particularly good at gaining respondent cooperation to attempt "refusal conversions." That is, these interviewers recontact individuals who refused a first interview attempt and make a second attempt to convince them to participate. If done well, this practice can raise response rates somewhat.

Quality of Completed Questionnaires

Supervisors should review completed questionnaires to be sure that interviewers are recording answers legibly, following skip patterns correctly, and recording answers that are complete enough for data entry. They should also look for evidence that interviewers are recording responses to open-ended questions verbatim rather than paraphrasing.

Another supervisory task is that of validating completed surveys—that is, confirming that the questionnaires were actually completed during interviews rather than simply filled out by interviewers. Although all survey researchers would like to believe that interviewers never falsify interviews, supervisors should do **validation checks** with a sample (about 10%) of respondents to make sure they recall having been interviewed and to ask about the interviewer's conduct. Example 6.22 displays a sample of a form that a supervisor might use for this task. As the example shows, the supervisor might repeat a few of the survey questions to see if the respondent's answers match the responses recorded by the interviewer. If the supervisor uses this technique, the repeated questions should be about information that does not change with time (e.g., birth date, height).

Knowing that supervisors will be doing periodic validations can help motivate interviewers to stick to the protocol. Survey researchers refer to in-person interviewers who par-

EXAMPLE 6.22
Sample Validation Callback Sheet

RESPONDENT'S NAME: _____
DATE OF INTERVIEW: _____
INTERVIEWER: _____

1. Was the interviewer on time? Courteous?

2. Did he/she hand you a map of your neighborhood at the beginning of the interview?

3. How long have you lived in that neighborhood?

4. What is your date of birth?

5. Did you feel you had enough time to answer the questions?

6. Do you have any questions or comments regarding the interview?

tially or completely falsify interview data as *curbstoners*—that is, they sit on curbstones to fill out interviews rather than ask respondents the questions. This practice, which is extremely unethical, poses a serious threat to the survey results. When curbstoners are discovered, surveyors will not usually permit them to continue working on a survey project in any capacity.

Validation checks may turn up some interviews that were not falsified, but were poorly done. In such cases, it is important for supervisors to provide feedback and additional training to the interviewers, and to monitor their performance closely for a time. If an interviewer cannot improve enough over a reasonable time period, he or she needs to be reassigned to a less demanding project or moved to a different task.

The data from interviews that are discovered to have been falsified or significantly incorrect are invalid and cannot be used. These interviews need to be repeated, if possible, and the rest of the offending interviewer's interviews must be checked and redone as necessary by another interviewer.

Quality of Interviewing

To determine how well an interviewer conducts interviews, the supervisor must observe some interviews directly. "High-quality" interviewing is interviewing in which appropriate introductions are made, questions are asked exactly as written, and probing is done appropriately and without bias. A supervisor may randomly accompany interviewers on respondent visits or may review audiotapes of interviews. By monitoring the quality of interviewers' work in this way, supervisors can give feedback to interviewers to keep quality and standardization high.

Another quality check carried out by supervisors has been mentioned above, that of editing every interview. Although interviewers are expected to edit each interview before submission, a supervisor or other designated reviewer (such as a more experienced interviewer) edits each interview again. The editor makes sure that the interviewer has used probes at the proper times, that the documentation is comprehensible and consistent with coded responses, and that responses do not seem to contradict each other. When the editor finds errors or inconsistencies, he or she gives feedback to the interviewer, often in the form of a written summary (see Example 6.23). The editor may also provide verbal feedback to the interviewer for purposes of retraining and reinforcement.

Editing a CAPI interview is a bit different from paging through a paper questionnaire. The editor does not have to go through the interview screen by screen to check the codes and notes; instead, the data from a computerized interview

EXAMPLE 6.23
Sample Editing Summary

ID Number: 123-45678
Editor: 217
Interview date: 11/17/2001
Edit Date: 11/27/2001

Editor's Checklist	Question (Q) #	Comments
Self-edit done (Yes/No)		
Wrong code entered by interviewer based on verbatim	Q E5 Coded 1 = (yes)	This question is asking about regular theatergoing for the past 2 years. According to the verbatim, the answer was yes only for the first year.
Unclear/ unreadable/ incomplete verbatim		
Probe not correctly recorded		
No probe when response unclear		
Indication of nonneutral probe		
General comments		

SOURCE: Center for Health Studies, Group Health Cooperative.

can be displayed on-screen or printed in summary form, as in Example 6.24. Each item has a "label"—that is, QA1 might be Question 1 in section A, ID1 might be the first field for the identification number, ID2 might be a second field for verification of the ID number, and so forth. The editor can scan the whole interview in this summary form and check to see if the codes match the text comments (in the case shown in Example 2.4, these are labeled "notes"). The editor should have a paper copy of the questionnaire at hand to look up the exact wording and response options for items being checked.

EXAMPLE 6.24
Sample CAI Summary Used for Editing

RESPONDENT NUMBER: 123-45678
Disposition: 0   Time: 17 minutes   Status: 9

RESTARTS: 1
   ID1: 123-45678
   ID2: 123-45678

INTDATE: 20011117

INTVTYPE: 5 METHOD: 4 CONTACT: 1 DESC1: 1
RISKBEN: 1   RISKBEN: 2

QA1: 19231021
QB2: 1   QC1: 5   QD1: 2   QE1: 1
QE2: 5   QE3: 2   QE4: 3   QE5: 1

-(note)- The 1st year I went to the theater a lot but I haven't been there in the last 8-12 months.

SOURCE: Center for Health Studies, Group Health Cooperative.

Comment: In this example, the editor knows that Question E5 asks about consistent theatergoing for the past 2 years, and that a code of 1 means yes (going con-

Example 6.24 continued

sistently for the entire 2 years). Because the verbatim note clearly indicates that the respondent has not been attending the theater in the past 8-12 months, the response should be no (in this case, a code of 5). If the respondent answered yes and then gave this statement, the interviewer should have probed for a clarification. The probes would be documented in the text note along with the respondent's additional clarifying comments. The interviewer should then have coded a 5.

INTERVIEWER SUPPORT

An important aspect of supervision is interviewer support. Interviewers need to feel that supervisors are their allies in the important process of accurate data collection, and that quality is valued above quantity (although a certain level of quantity must be maintained for cost-effectiveness). Supervisors need to be constructive in their feedback to interviewers and creative in offering solutions to problems encountered in the field. Above all, supervisors need to be *available* for timely feedback when questions arise and *prompt* in addressing larger problems that require input from expert members of the survey team (such as the investigators or the statistician) and must then be communicated to interviewers.

Supervisors should establish regular opportunities to demonstrate their support for the interviewers from the beginning of the project. They should schedule meetings (or conference calls, if interviewers are geographically dispersed) for regular updates and troubleshooting. They should be consistently available, by e-mail or telephone, to interviewers who may need quick questions answered.

To maintain standardization and provide backup for faulty human memories, supervisors also need to document in notes and minutes all ongoing survey team decisions about changes in survey protocol and other matters of importance and circulate this information to all interviewers. Even those who made particular decisions about protocol changes may have trouble recalling the details a year or two later when they need to describe the study's methods in a paper that is being written. Supervisors should be sure to file all notes and memos for easy access, because questions are likely to arise down the road.

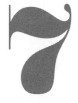

A Few Words About Managing and Analyzing Interview Data

This chapter briefly addresses the major tasks of data management and analysis in order to provide a complete picture of all of the steps involved in conducting survey interview research. For a more thorough discussion of these topics, see **How to Manage, Analyze, and Interpret Survey Data** (Volume 9 in this series). In the case of survey studies using in-person interviews, data management includes making sure that interviews done in the field make it to the survey center for editing, that the recorded answers are converted to a computer language suitable for analysis, and that the data are cleaned of any remaining identifiable errors. The survey team then analyzes the data—that is, performs the statistical procedures required to evaluate the survey's findings. As mentioned in Chapter 6, a parallel paper trail in the form of some type of control sheet or face sheet helps the surveyor to keep track of where interviews are in the path from data collection through analysis. The following checklist shows the tasks the surveyor must accomplish in carrying out data management and analysis. Each of these tasks is discussed briefly below.

Checklist of Data Management and Analysis Tasks

✓ Clean the data.

✓ Manage missing data.

✓ Plan the analysis.

✓ Analyze the data.

✓ Report on the data.

Cleaning the Data

The survey project's programmer will use a statistical program (such as SAS or SPSS) to check for "item-level" missing data (individual questions that were not answered), responses that do not fall into the range of possible answers, and other inconsistencies that may not be caught during the editing of the questionnaires. The programmer will also look for entire missing interviews, to see if they were lost or simply never completed. Whenever missing data can be filled in (after the interviewer and the respondent have been consulted) or answers that have obviously been miscoded can be corrected, the programmer can make these corrections directly in the database. This process of finding errors and correcting them is called *data cleaning*. Whenever corrections are made, they should be documented so that the reason for a change can be determined if confusion arises at some later time. Example 7.1 shows a sample of a table that might be used during data cleaning to document corrections to the database.

EXAMPLE 7.1
Sample Data Cleaning Table

Date Identified	ID#	Error	Date Cleaned
8/3/1999	91-123	Practice interview—delete entire interview.	8/12/1999
8/3/1999	92-534	Practice interview—delete entire interview.	8/12/1999
8/3/1999	91-425	Practice interview—delete entire interview.	8/12/1999
8/3/1999	93-012	Practice interview—delete entire interview.	8/12/1999
10/13/1999	93-178	H1 if R reports volunteer work, code "other" ("7") and specify.	1/5/2000
11/24/1999	91-127	G50.1 Trazodone is on list of antidepressants. It needs to be coded as "61," not "88."	2/16/2000
12/15/1999	91-451	F13. R's final verbatim says "no." The answer code should be "5," not "1."	2/16/2000
12/15/1999	93-617	H8. Owning their own business should be considered "self-employed" (code "2").	2/16/2000
1/13/2000	91-215	Wrong ID entered at ID 1 and 2. Should be 91-222.	1/21/2000
1/13/2000	92-192	Wrong ID at ID1. Should be 91-192. Check ID 2 and 3. Was intentionally done incorrectly b/c of problem above.	1/21/2000
2/10/2000	91-289	G39. This should be coded no, "5"—only paid counts, not family.	2/16/2000
2/10/2000	91-129	G39. This should be coded no, "5"—only paid counts, not family.	2/16/2000

SOURCE: Project IMPACT.

Managing Missing Data

When items are left blank or whole interviews are not done or lost, the first step is to try to get the data filled in by finding out if the interviewer forgot to record something or if the respondent can be called to answer the question(s). For data that cannot be filled in directly, surveyors sometimes employ a statistical procedure called *imputation,* which involves using a computer program to estimate the most likely response a respondent would have given, based, for example, on the answers of other similar respondents.

Planning the Analysis and Analyzing the Data

Once the data have been cleaned and the data from all interviews have been compiled into a complete database, a wide range of statistical analyses can be conducted. The surveyor and other users of the data will usually write an analysis plan in which they outline specific details to guide the programmer and statistician in setting up the proper calculations to answer specific questions. The analysis plan usually specifies (a) a particular research question to be answered, (b) the relevant sample (it could be the whole sample, just the female participants, only those who have had particular experiences, and so on), (c) which questionnaire items show the outcomes or results of interest (called dependent variables), (d) which items that may predict the outcomes of interest (called independent variables) are also to be examined, and (e) which statistical procedures are to be performed (e.g., chi-square analysis, logistic regression models). Programmers and statisticians write computer programs to perform the requested calculations and present the results to the survey team for interpretation.

Reporting on the Data

Once the numbers have been crunched, the survey team members consider the findings in light of the original research questions. They report their interpretations of the data to appropriate audiences through presentations and reports. Conclusions that are drawn from survey analyses may be used to drive decision making and may form the basis of scientific articles. The audience for the findings of a particular survey may be the board of directors of a company, a government committee attempting to make a funding decision, a group of scientists attending a scientific conference, or even the general public. Survey researchers can disseminate their findings very simply—for example, by sending memos to appropriate committee members—or they may develop formal reports, write articles for scholarly publications, or present papers orally in a variety of settings.

When a researcher formally reports on survey findings, the material is often presented in a common scientific format that divides the information into specific sections. The first is introductory information, or background material, often in the form of a literature review, in which the surveyor states what is already known about the topic and why the survey was done. Then the survey methods are spelled out in detail, including how the sample was obtained, how many people were sampled, how many refused to participate, what measures were included in the survey, and so on. Then the results are described in detail, but with little comment about their meaning. Finally, in the concluding section, the surveyor summarizes his or her interpretations of the findings, discusses the limitations of the survey's design, and may make recommendations for future studies.

The accuracy and interpretability of the survey findings that get reported rely heavily on the quality of the data collection procedures. Interviewers play a key role in collecting the data that lead to these important outcomes. The role of the interviewer in assuring valid and reliable data for such important interpretations should never be underestimated.

8 A Few Words About Qualitative Interviewing

 $\mathbf{B}$ ecause **qualitative interviewing** is often conducted in person, a brief discussion of this type of interviewing is called for in this book. For reasons that will be explained, qualitative methods are not often used for the kinds of surveys that are the subject of most of this volume and the others in this series. Qualitative methods have many useful applications, however, and can be used in combination with quantitative survey data collection techniques to broaden and enrich survey findings.

In qualitative interviews, the interviewer's interaction with the respondent is part of the data collection process. Such interviews are in-depth explorations in which respondents are encouraged to speak freely about whatever comes to mind regarding the interview topics. The interviewer takes notes and often tape-records the interview for later transcription, so that no detail is lost. Nonverbal gestures on the part of the respondent, body language, and any other phenomena that the interviewer notes may become part of the data. Although the interviewer is primarily a listener, he or she is not restrained by fully scripted response categories and pre-determined probes and prompts; the interviewer may usually ask clarifying questions as the situation warrants.

Researchers usually analyze the data from such interviews by organizing topics and themes that come up in the conversations and interpreting meanings conceptually rather than statistically. With the huge volume of data that can be collected in a single interview and a method of analysis that is based on cognitive insights rather than computations done by computer, the sample sizes in qualitative studies tend to be kept small. This form of interviewing is therefore not usually suited to the needs of large surveys. It is, however, a valuable research tool in general, and qualitative methods can be used to complement quantitative survey interviewing in a number of ways. For example, a study might be done to determine whether people who participate in a new education program are better able to quit smoking than others who participate in an existing program. A standardized interview can measure how many respondents in each group say they were able to quit, how hard they say the process was (on a scale of, say, *extremely hard* to *extremely easy*), and whether they believe the program they participated in was helpful. Statistics can then help determine whether the experience of the members of one group is *measurably* different from the experience of the members of the other—that is, in one group a larger proportion of people is counted who have quit smoking and who say they like the program. This may be important information for those who must decide whether the newer program should replace the existing one. But this method does not give the researcher conceptual insight into the actual experiences of the individual participants in the program, how they felt, and what subtle aspects worked well for them and why.

Even if such "what" and "why" questions are asked in the standardized survey, respondents are not usually able to report the level of conceptual detail that can be elicited by interviewers using qualitative methods. Some ideas might not even come to the respondent's mind in the context of the restricted questioning style required in a standardized interview. To address this, the surveyor might choose to do the standardized interview with a sample large enough to meet the statistical requirements of the study, and then ask a much smaller sample of these respondents to participate in qualitative interviews. In this smaller study, the surveyor can probe the nonquantifiable aspects of the respondents' experience with the smoking program.

There are many methods for conducting qualitative interviews, and they will not be detailed here. However, the following sections address some specific ways in which qualitative and quantitative interview research styles differ.

Interview Purpose and Goals

The purpose of qualitative interviewing is to describe and interpret experience, not to test hypotheses, find statistical differences between groups, or describe what proportion of a population holds a certain belief. Whereas quantitative methods may be used to test whether a hypothesis is true, qualitative methods are often used when there is not enough known for the researcher even to propose a hypothesis. In fact, the purpose of a qualitative interview may be to help generate hypotheses and ideas about a certain problem or question.

A variety of qualitative methods do not involve interviews at all; these include direct observation, the study of documents, and the study of videotaped interactions not involving the researcher. Like these other qualitative methods, qualitative interviews are aimed at getting at implicit aspects of experience to make them explicit. Qualitative researchers use interviews primarily to gather opinions, facts, and stories, and to gain insight into the experiences of others from the "inside."

Respondents

In any given qualitative study, interviews are usually done with only a few respondents (up to 50 or so, although larger samples have been reported). Statistical power is not a goal, and large samples cannot easily be analyzed with qualitative methods. Rather than asking a preselected sample of people the same set of questions, qualitative interviewers may simply continue interviewing people who have had the relevant experience until no new themes or ideas seem to be coming up anymore. And they often return to previous respondents to ask additional questions based on topics that have arisen during subsequent interviews. Respondent and interviewer have an interaction in which the respondent is not merely an object of study but a participant in the exploration of the research questions. After analysis, researchers often consult with their respondents to make sure that their descriptions of the findings accurately capture the respondents' experience.

Interviewers

Interviewers are an important part of the interview interaction in both quantitative and qualitative surveys. Although neutrality is important in the qualitative interview, in that the interviewer should not impose his or her own beliefs and interpretations on the exchange, the interviewer is engaged in the conversation, not just reading questions and recording responses as an interviewer would in a quantitative survey. Still, skilled interviewers need not say much during qualitative interviews—most of the talking is done by the respondents.

Interview Construction

As in quantitative survey studies, researchers conducting qualitative studies begin interview construction by defining the investigative objectives. The information elicited by the interviews must relate to the study's intent. Researchers often refer to the list of questions prepared for a qualitative interview as the *interview guide* (rather than the *questionnaire*). Although the goal is to get respondents to speak freely and in detail about each topic, interviewers do work from guides that bring some kind of order to the qualitative interview. Questions (or domains of interest not specifically stated as questions) are prepared and organized into a logical order. "Why" questions tend to be avoided, because they can make a respondent defensive. "Why" questions may be reframed as "what" or "how" questions that get at the same content. For example, "Why did you vote for that legislation?" could be reframed as "What considerations did you have in mind when you voted for that legislation?" or "How did you come to your decision about voting for this legislation?"

Qualitative interview guides may include a few probes and prompts that interviewers may use with respondents who are not saying much or do not seem to understand particular questions. Although qualitative interviews may not include many explicit questions, they can take a long time (often 2 to 3 hours or longer) as interviewers gather as much detail as possible.

Interview Administration

Although interviewers may use a casual approach to gain cooperation and put respondents at ease for qualitative interviews, their interview style is not haphazard. The questioning is deliberate, and the respondent should sense that there is a pace and rhythm to the encounter. The interviewer stays focused on the respondent and does not digress into personal stories and anecdotes. At the beginning of the interview, the interviewer states its general purpose as well as how long it is expected to take. As in quantitative interviews, the interviewer assures the respondent that all data will be treated with confidentiality; he or she may also describe the steps being taken to ensure confidentiality.

Often interviewers will tape-record qualitative interviews to make sure everything is captured (as in quantitative interviewing, respondent permission must be obtained for any such recording). Interviewers usually also take notes; this gives respondents time to think and shows them that what they are saying is being taken seriously.

During the qualitative interview, the interviewer pays careful attention. If responses on some topics seem incomplete, the interviewer has some freedom to refer back to them to encourage the respondent to say more. The interviewer does not have to repeat the original question verbatim, as in quantitative interviewing; he or she can be creative in finding ways to get the respondent to elaborate. For example, the interviewer might refer to statements made by others on the topic and then ask the respondent for reaction to those statements. Or the interviewer might speculate aloud: "I was wondering about this. Could it be that . . . ?"

At the end of the interview, the interviewer gives the respondent an opportunity to add any additional comments. The interview is closed with farewell pleasantries, and the interviewer explains that there is a possibility the respondent may be called on again to respond to new ideas that may come up and/or to confirm that the conclusions drawn from the interview seem accurate.

The environment of the qualitative interview is very important. Because the interviewer hopes to be accepted enough to gain an "inside" look at an experience, a certain comfort between the interviewer and respondent is necessary. The researcher needs to think in advance about the best places to conduct interviews, how interviewers should dress, and what gender and ethnic combinations in interviewer-respondent pairs are most likely to lead to open exchanges.

(Chapter 9 addresses the issue of cultural considerations in the survey interview environment.)

Coding

Because qualitative interviews are often used to generate new ideas and insights, precoding possible responses is usually impossible. For quantitative survey questions, surveyors can usually anticipate the range of likely answers, develop a list of answers, and number them in advance. The interviewer chooses the number of the answer provided, and the coding is complete (except for the data entry step if the interview is done on paper). Because questions for qualitative interviews are almost always open-ended, the data are usually in text form, either as detailed notes or as full interview transcripts prepared from tape recordings. The researcher might convert this text into codes developed after the interviews are done, or he or she may simply group statements and ideas according to themes that seem to be emerging from the data (without coding them).

Analysis

Researchers often use software programs that can assist them with the process of noticing recurring themes in text data and pointing out possible linkages between them. Users can code descriptive material into categories and even analyze it statistically to examine the occurrence of themes and their interrelations. Or a researcher may use the text data to develop hypotheses and theories by means of thorough examination of the meanings of the words in the texts. In qualitative analyses, it is the words that are interpreted; numbers are seldom involved. (For more information about content analysis for qualitative data, see **How to Manage, Analyze, and Interpret Survey Data,** Volume 9 in this series.)

Focus Groups

Aside from individual interviews, another useful qualitative interview method is the focus group. A **focus group** is a qualitative interview of several respondents at once; the surveyor is often interested in interactions within the group. The interviewer serves as moderator of the group, and the data produced are transcripts of the verbal exchanges among group members.

Focus groups can be used in conjunction with quantitative surveys in a number of ways. If a survey is to address a sensitive topic, for example, the surveyor may pretest some of the questions with a focus group to gauge how people might react: Are the questions understood in the way the surveyor intended them? Should the wording be modified? Sometimes a surveyor may not know at all how to conceptualize a topic in the form of survey questions and may form a focus group to help generate ideas. For example, a surveyor may seek to understand how to measure an abstract concept such as "confidence." To speculate about what factors may be associated with and predict high levels of confidence in individuals, the surveyor may conduct a focus group to find out how people spontaneously talk about this idea. From the themes that arise, he or she may develop ideas for questionnaire items that can later be assessed quantitatively. Perhaps a researcher is planning a survey that will measure respondent reaction to a tangible object, such as an educational booklet or a new toy. Conducting a focus group can help the researcher to anticipate the range of possible reactions to probe with the survey questions. Focus group feedback can also lead to refinement of the booklet or toy before it is presented to the larger target group.

Researchers can use focus groups to find out about the cross-cultural issues that may arise during interview administration in both quantitative and qualitative studies. The survey may target a particular cultural group or may be relevant to a mixed population in which more than one cultural context will be encountered. Rapport between interviewer and respondent, particularly during an in-person interview that may include the interviewer's spending time in the respondent's home, is very important. If the respondent sees the interviewer as an "outsider" who doesn't understand the respondent's cultural context, rapport, and therefore data quality, can be impaired. The respondent may not feel comfortable speaking candidly or may not expect the interviewer to understand his or her answers. Surveyors need to understand issues such as power differences between interviewer and respondent, differing nonverbal communication styles, variations in literacy levels and language use, and differing cultural taboos, especially those related to gender issues. Conducting focus groups can help survey researchers to anticipate issues that are relevant to particular cultural groups. Focus groups that are brought together for this purpose should probably include at least some bicultural members who can interpret the values and beliefs of the target group within the cultural contexts of the surveyor and interviewer.

The considerations noted above are among the larger ones that focus groups may help surveyors to understand before they send interviewers into the field. Focus groups may also uncover other issues, some of which may be quite subtle but highly useful to the surveyor in planning the project.

9 Cross-Cultural Considerations and Translations

Sensitivity to **cross-cultural issues** is important in the construction of interviews, both quantitative and qualitative, and must be considered in interviewer selection (age, gender, and cultural background) and training. In Latino cultures, for example, the interview relationship can be affected by "power distance," or the level of interpersonal power that exists between two individuals. Power is determined by certain characteristics of the individuals involved in an interaction, such as intelligence, wealth, social status, and age. A Latino respondent may see an interviewer as a powerful individual and may attempt to meet that person's expectations. In many cultures, demonstration of respect for persons of older age may be highly valued and can be an important concern for survey researchers who, for example, need to choose and train staff to interact with elderly participants.

In some cultures, the issue of protecting "face" is extremely important. The interviewer's attention to demonstrating respect and providing opportunities for the respondent to save face in the disclosure of personal information can be important in the interview relationship. Surveyors should also be aware of differences among cultures in expectations about "personal space" and orientation to time. For example, when a respondent arrives late for an interview, it may not be a reflection of how seriously he or she takes the commitment; rather, the respondent may come from a culture that is less strictly oriented to time than mainstream American culture.

In addition, surveyors should understand that what is perceived in one culture as an efficient, professional manner (e.g., the interviewer doesn't waste the respondent's time with too much small talk) may seem cold, distant, and impolite to individuals from another culture (where a bit of general banter may be seen as a sign of respect and genuine interest). Surveyors should also keep in mind the issue of gender differences. For example, in some cultures it may not be considered appropriate for a woman to be interviewed without her husband present, or for a female interviewer to be alone in a room with a male respondent.

Cross-cultural considerations lead to another obvious issue: How can survey researchers go about conducting interviews with immigrants who do not speak English at all, or with respondents in multiple countries where different languages are spoken? How can they make sure the questions in their survey instruments have the same meanings when translations are necessary?

Research has shown that it is often difficult to adapt questionnaires to cross-cultural contexts. For example, when a measure called the Nottingham Health Profile was translated into Arabic for use in Egypt, the resulting questionnaire items led to "embarrassment, disgust, horror, and accusations of blasphemy," according to one report. The importance of questionnaire translations that transcend the literal copying of meaning from one language to another has received significant attention. Experts in the field note the need for translated survey instruments to achieve semantic, idiomatic, experiential, and conceptual equivalence with the source documents. Survey researchers should view the translation of an instrument as having the same importance as the development of the original questionnaire.

Semantic equivalence refers to equivalence in the meaning of words between the original source and the translated version. Meaning is dependent on vocabulary and grammar. When a word can be interpreted in multiple ways and the word used in the translation captures only one of those meanings, or when grammatical forms used in the source document do not exist in the target language, it is difficult to preserve meaning or to use grammatically simple statements.

Idiomatic equivalence is important because idioms and colloquialisms are seldom similar across two languages. Concepts such as "feeling downhearted and blue" cannot be translated literally if the essential meaning of feeling depressed is to be preserved. In fact, literal translation of such a phrase would likely be humorous as well as meaningless. Equivalence of the information sought by a question, rather than equivalence of the wording, is what matters.

Experiential (or contextual) equivalence refers to the need to frame questions in terms of the experience of the respondent. For example, if members of the target group use the metric system, asking them to describe their consumption of soft drinks in ounces will result in unreliable answers, because measurements in ounces will be meaningless to them. Similarly, in a culture where respondents generally do not operate motor vehicles, it is probably pointless for a survey to include questions about drinking alcohol and driving.

Conceptual equivalence refers to the absence of differences in meaning and content between original and translated items. Words may be equivalent in semantic meaning but not in conceptual meaning. For example, in some cultures, drinking beer is not considered to be alcohol consumption, so respondents who drink only beer may answer no to a question asking if they drink alcohol, even when the word *alcohol* has been directly translated. In cultures where moderate consumption of alcohol is tolerated, the concept of feeling "guilty" after drinking alcohol may imply heavy consumption of alcohol, and so answers about such guilty feelings would be different from those the same questions might elicit in cultures where religious or cultural mores value abstention from alcohol, where even one drink may lead to feelings of guilt.

Response scales that assume a discrete meaning for each possible answer may also raise problems for a surveyor seeking conceptual equivalence between a translated version of a questionnaire and the original. For example, whereas an English-speaking respondent may understand the differences in the meanings of *excellent, very good,* and *good* and can choose among them to respond to a question (such as "How is your health?"), a Spanish-speaking respondent may consider direct translations of these words (*excelente, muy bien, bien*) to be equivalent in meaning. Repeating adverbs (e.g., *muy muy bien*) and using superlatives (e.g., *buenisimo*) may be better for distinguishing grades of meaning.

Perhaps the most encompassing aim of a translation is to achieve *cultural equivalence*. When the target language completely lacks a word or concept that is taken for granted in Western culture, translation becomes very challenging. Concepts of time, seasons, and moral standards, for example, vary from culture to culture. Questions involving such concepts may require very wordy translations; sometimes an item may need to be eliminated simply because it cannot be meaningfully rendered in the target language. Eliminated items may, in some cases, need to be replaced by completely new items.

In response to such important concerns, survey researchers have developed some methods for translating surveys and adapting them for cross-cultural use. Although these methods vary to some degree, most include some combination of the following steps:

1. *Multiple **translations** produced by more than one qualified translator:* It is recommended that translators be native speakers of the target language.

2. *Multiple **back-translations** (translations from the target-language version back to the original language) by translators who were not involved in the forward translation:* Back-translators should be native speakers of the original language of the questionnaire.

3. ***Committee review** to choose the best items generated among the various translations and to compare source and final versions:* It is recommended that this committee be made up of individuals from multiple disciplines, with bilingual and unilingual speakers of the target language, if feasible. This step sometimes involves a formal quantitative rating process to describe the conceptual equivalence of the translation with the back-translation or with the original version.

4. ***Lay panel review** to ensure the appropriateness of items for the specific audience of interest:* Translations made by highly educated individuals may be too literary or academic for the target audience (a phenomenon labeled the "posh effect" by the group translating the Nottingham Health Profile). Some authors recommend that this lay panel be made up of unilingual individuals, so that they cannot guess at items' original meanings.

5. ***Formatting** appropriate to the culture and language:* For example, the longer phrasing often necessary for Spanish translations may not fit the same formatting patterns used for the original version.

6. ***Pretesting** with a group of respondents sampled from the target population:* These respondents not only complete the instrument but are subsequently queried directly about their interpretations of the meaning of each item and its response options. Pretesting can also involve a reliability test using bilingual respondents answering both language versions of the questionnaire.

Translations conducted using variations and combinations of the methods listed above have produced "outwardly" equivalent questionnaires, even when the languages and cultures are rather distant from one another—such as English and Arabic, English and Cantonese, Laotian and Vietnamese—or when the instrument was translated into as many as 10 languages for a single project. That is, the questions were found to mean the same thing in all the languages. However, there is another kind of equivalence that surveyors must keep in mind: Because individuals from different cultures vary in their approaches to abstract concepts, questions designed to measure constructs (or concepts) in one language may not measure the same constructs in another. Surveyors can use various psychometric tests to determine whether the questions in a scale seem to measure the same thing in all language versions of the questionnaire.

When a survey involves translations, there are obvious implications for the selection and training of interviewers. Bilingual and/or bicultural interviewers, when they can be found, may have an easier time understanding and bridging cultural differences, although training can help many interviewers to overcome some barriers even if the interviewers do not share the respondents' cultural background. Clearly, the interviewer must have excellent command of the language of the interview, not only to deliver the questions properly, but also to understand the nuances in the meanings of respondents' answers. Interviewers also need to be fluent enough in the language of the interview to make general conversation with respondents, both to enhance rapport and to dispel any discomfort respondents may feel about admitting a stranger into the home or revealing sensitive information.

Interviewers need to receive training concerning culturally appropriate (and inappropriate) behaviors as well as linguistic issues that may apply to specific questions in one language but not another. For example, probes and prompts for particular questions may need to vary from one language to the next. Some questions may be entirely different in one language versus another, and yet measure the same content. These differences need to be made clear in the Q by Qs, and interviewers need to study them during training. Supervisors need to make significant efforts to bring interviewers together regularly to exchange stories about their experiences and share the challenges they have encountered in administering the interview. This will allow the survey team to identify inadvertent departures from standardized methods and will enhance the interpretation of survey findings within a rich understanding of the cultural context of each language version.

Exercises

1. List the factors that you should consider in determining whether in-person interviewing is the best mode of administration for a given survey.

2. You have been funded to do a survey of 1,000 elementary school teachers' opinions of the quality of education in your state. You anticipate that 30-minute in-person interviews will be done using CAPI at 50 schools across the state. The schools are located within five geographic regions. You have designed sampling procedures for selecting teachers from within each school in advance of the interviews. You have a year to complete the interviews, and data analysis and reporting will occur in the second year. What are the factors you should consider in setting up an administrative plan for this survey?

3. You need to ask respondents how much sugar-free soda they consume in a week. You determine that soda is most commonly packaged in 16-ounce cans, 20-ounce bottles, and 2-liter bottles. A 2-liter bottle contains about 8.5 8-ounce servings. You have also researched the most common sizes of cups for fountain drinks. Describe a visual aid you might use to help respondents estimate how much soda they drink in a week.

4. For each of the following scenarios, name the question-order effect that is operating and state how this problem might be overcome.

   a. An interview has been going on for 45 minutes. A complex question is next, and it may be hard for the respondent to catch all of the details if it is read by the interviewer. Instead, the interviewer hands the respondent a card on which is printed a long paragraph about pesticide use in a nearby agricultural area. The respondent skims the card quickly, so the interviewer offers to read the material aloud after all. The respondent says, "No, I understand it. What's the question?" The interviewer reads the question and four response options to the respondent. The respondent answers, "Uh, the first one, I guess." The interviewer starts to repeat the options. The respondent says, "It's the first one. Let's just keep going."

   b. Near the beginning of an interview, the respondent is asked whether he considers consumption of salty snacks to be unhealthful. The respondent answers yes, extremely unhealthful, and adds that he has heard from a doctor that salt is bad for you and that many salty snacks are also high in fat. Later in the interview, the respondent is asked to estimate his consumption of specific types of salty snacks in the past month. The respondent hesitates a lot and tends to indicate low consumption levels.

   c. At the beginning of an interview, the respondent is asked how often she exercises for leisure during a typical month. A later question is part of a series of questions about behaviors the respondent specifically engages in to promote health. The question is fifth in a series of seven and reads, "How often do you exercise during a typical month?" The respondent is irritated and says, "Like I said before, about three times."

5. You are doing a door-to-door survey, and a potential respondent tells you he is not interested in participating before you have even finished describing it. How might you respond?

6. A woman from another culture is to be interviewed about her attitudes concerning parenting. What factors should the survey team consider in preparing for the interview and in setting up the space for the interview?

7. You are a supervisor for a large survey project and one of your interviewers cannot get the hang of the procedures for uploading completed interviews to the project Web site. There is a danger that interviews will be destroyed or lost. How might you respond to this problem?

8. You are about to send a team of newly trained interviewers into the field to perform a survey using laptop computers. They will be carrying their materials with them to respondents' homes. Design a "handy reminders" checklist to help them make sure they have everything they need on hand.

9. You are conducting a large-scale survey at 10 sites across the country. A section of the interview asks about the respondent's use of contraceptives and general attitudes toward the use of contraceptives. You recognize that this may be a sensitive subject, especially within certain subgroups.

   a. Describe some ways to deal with the sensitive topic within the structure of the interview.

   b. Suggest a way in which you can explore how the

subject may be perceived in different subgroups in advance, so that you can use the information to inform the design and wording of survey questions.

ANSWERS

1. Factors that you should consider in deciding whether in-person interviewing is the most appropriate mode of survey administration for a particular project include the following:

   - *Type of respondent:* Are in-person interviews more appropriate because respondents are likely to be hard of hearing, too young to be interviewed over the phone or to fill out questionnaires on their own, or difficult to access by telephone or mail?

   - *Complexity of the questionnaire:* Are the questions complex, or are there long lists of response options? Are there confusing aspects of the questionnaire that are best dealt with using visual aids and that require some probing and prompting by a well-trained interviewer?

   - *Length of the interview:* Is the questionnaire long enough that the presence of an interviewer will be advantageous in keeping the respondent involved?

   - *Nature of the questions:* Are the questions mostly of a kind that could be influenced by the presence of an interviewer? That is, might they cause the respondent to answer less honestly for fear of offending or putting off the interviewer? Might the respondent be embarrassed to answer honestly in front of an interviewer?

- *Sampling needs:* Does the research question require a scientific sample with a high response rate, or will a less complete sample suffice?

- *Cost:* Is there enough funding available for the survey to be done well using in-person interviewing?

2. You will need to evaluate a great many factors in planning the survey. Following are some of the main issues requiring attention:

   - *Space:* You will need to set up a location (a survey center) for receiving, cleaning, analyzing, and storing data. You must consider also how this space needs to be furnished (chairs, desks, computers, filing cabinets).

   - *Personnel:* You will need to identify individuals who will be responsible for setting up procedures, training interviewers, programming the analysis, and so on.

   - *Equipment:* You will need to think about how many computers will be needed, both for the survey center and in the field.

   - *Training:* You will need to consider how much interviewer training will be required and where it will take place. For example, will all training be done centrally at the survey center, or will trainers travel to each site in the field?

   - *Questionnaire development:* You will need to consider many issues as you develop the questionnaire. For example: Who contributes questions? How will the instrument be pretested? When does a working draft need to be ready for training?

   - *Data tracking procedures:* You will need to plan how data tracking will be handled. For example: How will interviewers turn in their interviews? How often will they submit batches? What forms will be needed for tracking interviews from the field through data entry and data cleaning?

- *Data management:* You will need to have a data management plan: Who will edit completed interviews? How will data cleaning be documented?

- *Confidentiality:* You must consider what the confidentiality requirements of the survey will be. Will IRB approval be required? How will confidentiality be assured?

- *Analysis and dissemination:* You will need to plan for both analysis of the data and dissemination of the survey findings. Who do you need to consult with to make sure the data will answer the research questions at the analysis stage? What reports will be required, what decisions will depend on these findings, and when will they be due?

3. You could create a card with drawings depicting all of the common types of soda containers, with the number of ounces each container holds printed next to the appropriate drawing. Respondents could then be asked how many of each type of container of soda they consume, on average, in a week. You could allow respondents to make estimates of partial amounts (such as half of a 2-liter bottle).

4. a. This is the *fatigue effect.* The respondent is bored and wants to get done with the interview. Whenever possible, it is wise to place complex questions early in the interview, after rapport has been established but before the respondent has become tired.

   b. This is the *consistency effect.* The respondent may be trying to bring his consumption answers into consistency with his view that eating salty snacks is unhealthy. It may be better to ask the consumption question first.

c. This is the *redundancy effect*. The two questions seem too similar for the respondent to recognize that one pertains to leisure activities and the other to exercise specifically for health improvement. The difference can be made more explicit in the wording of the questions, and the interviewer can use prompts to help the respondent recognize the difference. The interviewer can also acknowledge the apparent redundancy and explain that although it may not be obvious, there are reasons the questions are organized in this way, and the respondent's answers to both questions are very helpful.

5. You might mention how important it is to talk to everyone in the sample and how important this specific individual's responses are for the survey. You can also make assurances about confidentiality that may put the person more at ease. If there doesn't seem to be any chance of saying more about what the survey is about, let it go. Acknowledge that this may be a bad time and offer to come back or have a colleague come back or call at a better time.

6. It is important to consider the interviewer-respondent match. Will an interviewer's age or gender influence how the respondent feels about discussing her personal opinions about parenting? How much interpersonal space is appropriate in the respondent's culture? Is it appropriate to make eye contact? How can you assure privacy so that other caregivers and children are not in the background during the interview, possibly affecting how comfortable the respondent feels in giving honest answers? Also consider how the interviewer should dress for the interview. Will the interviewer's dressing too formally create separation between the interviewer and respondent in a way that could affect responses? Will the interviewer's dressing too casually cause the respondent not to take the interview seri-

ously or to feel disrespected? You need to consider all these questions in the context of the respondent's culture.

7. Be supportive and creative. Provide additional training right away. It is probably necessary to have a supervisor or experienced interviewer (either physically present or on the phone) walk the interviewer through the process a few times, supported by a set of written instructions. Troubleshoot until the interviewer catches on. Make sure the interviewer makes backup copies of all interviews before attempting to upload, in case anything goes wrong.

8. The following are some of the items you might include on a reminder list:

   - Laptop computer (make sure battery is charged)

   - Extra charged battery

   - Cell phone (make sure battery is charged)

   - Enrollment form (if used and not already filled out)

   - Consent forms (extra copy to give to respondent after signature)

   - Incentive gift (if used)

   - Diskettes to back up interview files

   - Paper survey (in case the computer fails)

   In addition, you might add a note at the end of the list reminding the interviewer to edit each interview as soon as possible after completion.

9. a. You can deal with a sensitive topic by placing the question well into the interview so that rapport has been established between the interviewer and respondent before the question is asked. Another possibility is to place the sensitive questions on a separate page so the interviewer can hand the page

to the respondent to be filled out privately. The interviewer should be sure to give the respondent assurances of complete confidentiality.

b. You could conduct several focus groups, each made up only of members of one of the various subgroups, to explore reactions to the subject in advance.

Suggested Readings

Atkinson, R. (1998). *The life story interview*. Thousand Oaks, CA: Sage.

Gives specific guidelines for preparing, administering, and interpreting life-story interviews.

Converse, J. M., & Presser, S. (1986). *Survey questions: Handcrafting the standardized questionnaire*. Beverly Hills, CA: Sage.

Provides a brief but excellent discussion of question writing and administration.

Converse, J. M., & Sherman, H. (1974). *Conversations at random: Survey research as interviewers see it*. New York: John Wiley.

Classic account of how interviewers perceive the task of interviewing, especially how they overcome respondent resistance and how a standardized list of questions is administered in somewhat unstandardized contexts.

Fowler, F. J., Jr., & Mangione, T. W. (1990). *Standardized survey interviewing: Minimizing interviewer-related error*. Newbury Park, CA: Sage.

Discusses recruiting, training, and supervision of interviewers, techniques of asking questions, and strategies for interviewers to use in establishing working relationships with respondents. The major focus is on reducing errors that might be attributed to the interviewing process.

Frey, J. H. (1989). *Survey research by telephone* (2nd ed.). Newbury Park, CA: Sage.

Review of sampling, questionnaire construction, question writing, and interviewing associated with telephone interviews. Includes an extensive chapter comparing telephone, mail, in-person, and intercept surveys on several dimensions, such as costs, response rates, and data quality.

Frey, J. H., & Fontana, A. (1991). The group interview in social research. *Social Science Journal, 28,* 175-187.

Review of the various formats for group interviews that have been used in research settings. Both casual, informal field situations and formal, controlled contexts are conducive to this type of interview.

Gorden, R. L. (1987). *Interviewing: Strategy, techniques, and tactics* (4th ed.). Homewood, IL: Dorsey.

Extensive discussion of the factors that influence the dynamics of in-person interviewing. Discusses the appropriate setting for interviews and how interviewers must deal with verbal and nonverbal communication in the interview context.

Gorden, R. L. (1992). *Basic interviewing skills.* Itasca, IL: Peacock.

Excellent review of all stages of the interview, from designing relevant questions to establishing a proper atmosphere for interviewing, listening to the respondent, probing responses, and properly recording information.

Groves, R. M., & Kahn, R. L. (1979). *Surveys by telephone: A national comparison with personal interviews.* New York: Academic Press.

One of the first studies to compare telephone and in-person interviews on a variety of dimensions, including sampling, response rates, item nonresponse, cost, and response error. Includes an important comparison of random-digit dialing sampling design with area probability designs.

Gubrium, J. F., & Holstein, J. A. (Eds.). (2002). *Handbook of interview research: Context and method.* Thousand Oaks, CA: Sage.

Excellent resource containing a broad collection of essays on various aspects of interview research. Provides expert discussions of conceptual and methodological issues related to forms of interviewing, distinctive respondents, use of technology, and analytic strategies.

Hendricson, W. D., Russell, I. J., Prihoda, T. J., Jacobson, J. M., Rogan, A., & Bishop, J. D. (1989). An approach to developing a valid Spanish language translation of a health-status questionnaire. *Medical Care, 27,* 959-966.

Useful article detailing methodological issues pertaining to translations.

Holstein, J. A., & Gubrium, J. F. (1995). *The active interview.* Thousand Oaks, CA: Sage.

Helpful guidebook for those who use qualitative methods. Describes the differences between an active interview and the traditional interview and provides a basis for rethinking interview procedures.

Hunt, S. M. (1986). Cross-cultural issues in the use of socio-medical indicators. *Health Policy, 6,* 146-158.

Describes issues that arise from the translation of existing questionnaires and details the practical problems arising specifically from the translation of the Nottingham Health Profile into Arabic and Spanish.

Hunt, S. M., Alonso, J., Bucquet, D., Niero, M., Wicklund, I., & McKenna, S. (1991). Cross-cultural adaptation of health measures. *Health Policy, 19,* 33-44.

Describes technical, linguistic, and conceptual issues raised by the translation of existing measures from English into other languages.

Hyman, H. H., et al. (1955). *Interviewing in social research.* Chicago: University of Chicago Press.

Good review of interviewing principles. Includes a particularly important discussion of the impact of interviewer expectations.

Kirk, J., & Miller, M. L. (1985). *Reliability and validity in qualitative research.* Newbury Park, CA: Sage.

Discusses objectivity in qualitative research and the problems of validity and reliability, as well as ethnographic decision making.

Marin, G., & Marin, B. O. (1991). *Research with Hispanic populations.* Newbury Park, CA: Sage.

Excellent resource concerning cross-cultural considerations researchers should take into account when working with Hispanic populations.

McCracken, G. (1988). *The long interview.* Newbury Park, CA: Sage.

Provides comprehensive coverage of the methods and issues involved in intensive qualitative interviewing.

Morgan, D. L. (Ed.). (1993). *Successful focus groups: Advancing the state of the art.* Newbury Park, CA: Sage.

Anthology includes contributions from leading authorities in the use of group interviewing, especially focus groups, in research. Clearly delineates the advantages and disadvantages of this type of research. Includes several accounts of how the group interview can be used to augment survey implementation.

Morgan, D. L. (1996). *Focus groups as qualitative research* (2nd ed.). Thousand Oaks, CA: Sage.

Discusses focus groups as a qualitative method, uses of focus groups, how to design and conduct focus groups, and analysis of focus group data for research in every discipline.

Morgan, D. L., & Krueger, R. A. (1997). *The focus group kit* (6 vols.). Thousand Oaks, CA: Sage.

Comprehensive series provides guidance on planning, developing questions for, and moderating focus groups, as well as involving community members in focus groups.

Oppenheim, A. N. (1992). *Questionnaire design, interviewing, and attitude measurement.* New York: St. Martin's.

Excellent discussion of the issues of survey design, with especially valuable chapters on pilot studies, attitude measurement, and the characteristics of standardized interviewing.

Rossi, P. H., Wright, J. D., & Anderson, A. B. (Eds.). (1983). *Handbook of survey research.* San Diego, CA: Academic Press.

Comprehensive and detailed review of all aspects of survey design, including sampling theory, measurement issues, survey administration, computerization, and data analysis. Chapters by Bradburn on response effects and Sheatsley on questionnaire construction and item writing offer excellent discussions.

Schuman, H., & Presser, S. (1981). *Questions and answers in attitude surveys: Experiments on question form, wording, and context.* New York: Academic Press.

Uses more than 30 national surveys conducted over a 6-year period to compare open versus closed formats, wording strategies, question-order effects, and response-order variations.

Glossary

Advance letter (or preletter)—Letter sent to a potential respondent to introduce a survey for which the individual may be eligible to participate. The preletter serves to authenticate the survey and gives the respondent time to think about participating before he or she is contacted by telephone or in person.

Back-translation—The rendering of translated documents (such as interview scripts) back into their original language. Back-translation, which should be done by a person other than the person who did the original translation, is used to assess whether the source document was accurately captured by the initial translation.

Computer-assisted interviewing (CAI) software—Software that is used to program interviews for computer administration.

Computer-assisted personal interviewing (CAPI)—Interviewing conducted by an interviewer using a computer (usually a laptop) in the physical presence of the respondent. The interviewer reads the questions and response options from the computer screen and records responses directly into the computer.

Confidentiality—Protection of a respondent's identity as a participant in a survey or study. Rules of confidentiality require that survey researchers not reveal the names of respondents, or their addresses or other identifying information, to anyone except as required by law. Materials containing identifiers are safeguarded by all reasonable means, including storage in locked areas.

Consistency effect—A question-order effect that arises when respondents feel that their answers to particular questions must be consistent with their answers to previous questions.

Cross-cultural issues—Cultural factors that may have impacts on the relationship between interviewer and respondent. Surveyors need to consider cultural differences in gender taboos, acceptable interpersonal space, attitudes toward age, orientation to time, and other factors in preparing an interview, and interviewers need to be aware of cultural differences in order to administer the interview sensitively.

Data entry—The step of entering codes for interview responses into a computer for analysis.

Double-barreled question—An interview question that asks two things at once. Such questions are confusing to the respondent, and the responses are difficult to analyze, because it is unclear which part of such questions the respondent has answered.

Editing—The process of reviewing the questionnaire after the interview is completed to look for and correct errors and make clarifications. Interviewers should always edit completed questionnaires before submitting them; second edits should be carried out by supervisors or other project staff.

Eligibility screen—A set of questions designed to screen out potential respondents who do not meet the criteria of characteristics and/or experiences necessary for participation in a particular survey.

Fatigue effect—A question-order effect in which respondents' attention to and interest in the interview decrease as they become weary or bored. Respondents who are fatigued may stop answering thoughtfully.

Focus group—A carefully selected group of people who are brought together to give their opinions and offer their perspectives on specific topics. Questioning is conducted as a group interview in which individual responses as well as group interaction are part of the data collected.

Informed consent—Consent given by respondents certifying that they are participating with full knowledge of the risks and benefits of participation, the activities that constitute participation, the terms of participation, and their rights as research subjects.

Interviewer—A trained individual who asks the survey's scripted questions and records respondents' answers on the questionnaire (whether on paper or in a computer).

Interviewer effect—Bias introduced into respondents' answers to interview questions caused by factors related to the presence of the interviewer. Respondents may answer less honestly than they would on a self-administered survey, or they may be influenced by an interviewer's appearance, gender, or age to answer questions in a certain way.

Loaded question—An interview question that implies a preferred response; such questions are often emotional in tone and should be avoided.

Pilot test—A full "dress rehearsal" of the survey project, performed to see if the questionnaire and the various project procedures will work as envisioned.

Precall—A telephone call made to a potential respondent to introduce a survey for which he or she may be eligible. The precall serves to authenticate the survey and give the respondent time to think before further contact is made.

Pretesting—Testing of the interview questionnaire under "mock" conditions to see whether question wording and transition statements are adequate, to find out how long the average interview may take, and to get a sense of any problems that may exist with the interview itself.

Probe—A technique used by the interviewer to obtain more information if a respondent's answer is unclear, irrelevant, or incomplete. Probes may or may not be verbal. An interviewer may probe simply by pausing, by repeating the question or the respondent's reply, or by asking a neutral question.

Prompt—A predetermined statement used by the interviewer when the respondent seems confused or unclear about how to answer a question. Interviewers should be trained to use standard neutral prompts as necessary. When a question is expected to require a detailed specific prompt, it is written into the questionnaire for the interviewer to read verbatim if needed.

Qualitative interviewing methods—Interviewing methods used by researchers who are concerned with uncovering meanings. In qualitative survey studies, the interaction between the interviewer and respondent is intended to get at deeper levels of meaning on the subject of study. Results are analyzed conceptually.

Quantitative interviewing methods—Interviewing methods used by researchers who are concerned with measurement. Quantitative methodology requires that survey administration be standardized to minimize variation from interview to interview. Results are analyzed statistically.

Question-by-question specifications (Q by Qs)—A list that explains the purpose of every question in an interview and provides the interviewer with clarification of any confusing aspects of each question and any important coding instructions.

Questionnaire—The script used for a survey. Interview questionnaires include the questions and response options; transition statements; instructions to the interviewer for skipping, probing, and prompting; and any other instructions necessary for smooth administration of the interview.

Recommended responses (or fallback statements)—Standardized answers that interviewers are instructed to give to common general questions asked by respondents, such as questions pertaining to the nature of the interview, who is sponsoring the work, and what participation will entail. Interviewers are instructed to learn the responses and keep the printed version handy for reference as necessary.

Redundancy effect—A question-order effect that occurs when questions seem to be repeating previous questions; when this happens, respondents may not answer carefully, if at all. Sometimes redundancy in the questionnaire is intentional or cannot be avoided for methodological reasons. Interviewers need to read all questions carefully, so that respondents can sense differences in meaning. When redundancy is required, interviewers can make neutral statements that acknowledge the repetition and ask that the respondent please answer again.

Refusal conversion—An attempt to change a potential respondent's mind when he or she has refused to participate in an interview. Usually, experienced interviewers are assigned to recontact "refusers" and politely attempt to "convert" them to agreeing to participate.

Respondent—An individual who provides answers to survey questions.

Response options—Predetermined choices from which respondents select their answers (e.g., five choices ranging from 1 = *strongly agree* to 5 = *strongly disagree*).

Response rate—The proportion of eligible respondents who actually complete the interview. If there are a large number of refusals, the response rate will be low, making the survey's results less meaningful.

Skip pattern—An instruction to the interviewer regarding how to move through the questionnaire depending on the respondent's answers. For example, "If the answer to question 1 is yes, continue with question 2. If the answer is no, skip to question 7." Skipping instructions are printed on the page in paper questionnaires. In CAPI, the computer does the skipping automatically.

Socially desirable response—An answer that a respondent gives because he or she thinks it is the "politically correct" response or what the interviewer wants to hear (rather than what the respondent really thinks).

Standardization—The process of keeping variations in interview administration to a minimum so that every respondent hears the same questions and response choices and is not influenced by the interviewer's perspective.

Survey—A system for collecting information from or about people to describe, compare, or explain their knowledge, attitudes, and behavior. In-person interviews are one method for collecting survey information.

Transition statement—A statement within the questionnaire that introduces a new topic, separates topic sections, or announces a change in format (such as a new response set). The interviewer reads all transition statements to the respondent as written.

Validation check—A procedure in which an interviewing supervisor recontacts a respondent to confirm that the interview was carried out correctly, usually by repeating certain interview questions (questions for which the answers would not have changed over time, such as birth date). Validation checks may reveal falsified interviews and poor interviewing practices.

About the Author

Sabine Mertens Oishi holds an M.S.P.H. degree in epidemiology from the University of California, Los Angeles. She is currently the project manager of the UCLA-based coordinating center for Project IMPACT, a multisite national study evaluating a care model for late-life depression using in-person and telephone interviewing. She has been a researcher with Arlene Fink Associates, Pacific Palisades, California, where she was involved in program evaluations of health and social services programs and health professional training programs. She has participated in a variety of research projects at UCLA, RAND, and the Veterans Administration Medical Center in Sepulveda, California. As a Peace Corps volunteer, she participated in the implementation of an in-person knowledge, attitude, and practice survey for diarrheal disease in urban and rural Liberia, West Africa, in collaboration with the Liberian Ministry of Health and Social Welfare, U.S. Peace Corps, and USAID.